Where to Go When You're Hurting:
A Healing Resource Guide

by Elizabeth Rosenthal, MPH, MBA, Ph.D.

To Holly,

A fellow traveler.

With all my love,

Beth
3/98

Where to Go When You're Hurting:
A Healing Resource Guide

EMPR
P.O. Box 14684, Chicago, IL 60614-0684

© 1998 Elizabeth Rosenthal

Chapter 4, Definitions of Treatments, written
by Health Care Futures.

Cover Illustration: Vanessa Vermond

Book Design and Layout: Jar Design

Publisher's Cataloging-in-Publication
(Provided by Quality Books, Inc.)

Rosenthal, Elizabeth A., 1963 -
    Where to go when you're hurting : a healing resource
guide / by Elizabeth Rosenthal. -- 1st ed.
    p. cm.
    Includes bibliographical references and index.
    ISBN: 0-9660472-0-6

    1. Holistic medicine--Directories. 2. Alternative
medicine--Directories. 3. Healing. I. Title.

R733.R67 1998   362.1'78
                           QBI98-54

First Printing
10 9 8 7 6 5 4 3 2 1

DISCLAIMER

This publication is designed to provide accurate and authoritative information with regard to the subject matter covered. It is sold with the understanding that the publisher is not engaged in rendering legal, accounting, or other professional advice. If legal advice or other expert assistance is required, the services of a competent professional person should be sought.

▼

The resources listed in this book have not been screened. Neither the author or publisher guarantee the accuracy of the information provided. Although every attempt has been made to provide accurate information, we do not assume responsibility for listings included or omitted from this book. You are responsible for investigating providers before you use them, and the search for healing practices and providers is often in itself an important part of the healing process. We offer you these resources along with our best wishes for exploring your health options.

To arrange speaking and consulting engagements with Dr. Rosenthal, order books, submit resources to be listed in the guide or put yourself on the mailing list, use the forms at the end of the book, or contact her at:

EMPR
P.O. Box 14684, Chicago, IL 60614-0684
(773) 348-8248
(888) 302-8248
E-mail: drbeth@ibm.net
www.healthy-solutions-us.com

ACKNOWLEDGMENTS

I acknowledge and thank my parents, Lynne and Mason Rosenthal, who have supported me in every way possible. There are no two people who could have been more ideal parents.

For the gifts they have given me, I thank: David, Tom, Jian, and Ted Rosenthal; Leo Guthman; the late Cecile Guthman; Andrea Burleson; Don Eisenstein; Laurence Mulliez-Hurel; Anna-Lisa Espinoza; Nancy Latham; and Mark Gusho.

The Definitions of Treatments chapter was written by Mary Ann Neis, R.N., M.N. and Barbara Manley-Wheeler, R.N., M.S. of Health Care Futures. Their organization provides workshops, consultations, and lectures about complementary, or alternative, medicine. It has been a pleasure working with these committed individuals. Contact information for Health Care Futures is listed in Section I of the Resource Listing under the educational organization/program heading.

Remaining Thanks

Karen Alberg Grossman, a friend of many, many years did a superb job of editing - the remaining flaws are entirely mine.

Pauline Russell, a woman of abundance and possibility, propelled this book into existence and lights me up with her being. I could not have had a better marketing and public relations person.

Roan Kaufman, a treasure of friendship, support, straight talk and laughs, graciously took care of all my pre-press concerns.

Vanessa Vermond, an extraordinary artist, blessed me with her exuberance and the cover design of my dreams.

Tem Horwitz, a very gifted and generous T'ai Chi teacher, philosopher, and life guide, strengthened and nurtured my chi whenever I most needed it.

Roni Ambrister, co-founder of Women In Spiritual Evolution (WISE Women) gave me valuable comments on an early draft.

Sonia Choquette recognized my mission before I did, and gave me the clarity and courage to pursue it.

Dr. George Zabrecky provided me with my first glimpses of good health. It was in his presence that this book was conceived.

I acknowledge the transformational human beings who participate in the work of Landmark Education Corporation and are creating worlds of possibilities.

And finally, thanks go to all who spent time with me talking about this book, and provided guidance and resources.

Introduction by Pauline Russell

Beth Rosenthal and I met in 1996 in a training and development program about breakthrough thinking. At that time what I knew of Beth was that she was working on completing her Ph.D. at the University of Chicago in business management. What I didn't know was that she was writing a book – the one you are reading now – that would change my life and beliefs about what it is to be well forever.

Almost one year later in August of 1997 we, along with 600 other people, were at another program in Los Angeles, California. Before the weekend seminar began I was relaxing by the pool reading the final draft of the book. There were two new chapters that I had not read in earlier drafts. I was reading these chapters, not only as her public relations and marketing person, but as someone who suffered from migraines starting from age 12, around my first period. I looked in the index for headaches or migraines. Neither was listed. Before dinner I asked Beth why neither were listed. She explained that one should look at health as a total picture and treat the whole person – mind, body and spirit – not just individual symptoms. That was not exactly what I wanted to hear, but as I completely trust Beth, I listened.

Two days later I had my period and a migraine so severe I couldn't see or hear. The pain was so bad I kept sticking things – the tip of my pen, my fingers, my water bottle, the alarm clicker for the rental car – into the small crevice between the bridge of my nose and the corner of my eye where the pain and pressure seemed to start. Everyone in our group could see I was in terrible pain and bad shape. The prescription medicine was not working.

Beth talked to me about going up to the room and lying down. What she said to me was something I had never believed before: that it was okay to have the headache and take care of myself. Being sick did not equal being a bad person. Although I was in charge of my well-being I wasn't wrong or bad because I was sick.

When I got into bed I cried. Being sick to me was wrong. Sickness was a sign of weakness and failure. If you were ill there was something for which you were not taking responsibility. Or you were doing something wrong with regard to your health. I was angry, frustrated and disgusted with myself for being sick! The next day my friends and colleagues had conversations about my migraines – what I could be doing to stop having them. I was extremely frustrated. For twenty-two and a half years I've heard about this cure or that cure for migraines and I feel as though I've tried them all.

The breakthrough I had from reading this book and being with Beth is that wellness is a journey and there is NOTHING WRONG WITH ME! Wellness is a building process like building a house. First you start with an idea or commitment, and then you create a blueprint. Then you build a foundation, and then add a frame and a roof, then paint and finally decorate with furniture, artwork, books, and so on to create a space that is yours.

Beth Rosenthal's commitment and the promise of this book is two fold: First, for people to understand that being ill is not their fault. And second, to empower people on their journey for well-being.

One last note – you are perfect as you are! This resource guide is a road map in your adventure for creating your own well-being.

Pauline Russell

Chicago, August 1997

1

CHAPTER ONE: LIVING A LIFE IN BALANCE

This book is an expression of love and hope. Finding the kind of health care that works best and is most comfortable for you is important whether you are sick and wanting to feel better or healthy and wanting to stay that way. Health care should be respectful and compassionate, as well as empowering. The power of healing often lies within us, and we can learn how to access it. No one should have to contend with limited, non-compassionate health care. There are many choices available and knowing what the options are and how to access them is an important component of healing.

Doing what we know is good for us isn't always easy. I myself am a chocoholic, so I tend to each much more chocolate than is good for me. Some people don't get enough sleep, work too much, drink too much, or, at the other extreme, are fanatical about eating only healthy foods or adhere to rigid, overly disciplined exercise regimes. Both extremes reflect unbalanced lives. Living a life in balance isn't easy. I offer my experiences in trying to live a life in balance as example and encouragement. I talk about some of the health choices I've made and how I incorporate them into my lifestyle. This book is also a resource guide about the integration of holistic and conventional medicine. There are hundreds of resources listed to help you find what is right for you, and suggestions for how to find the right practice, practitioner, or program.

While there is a growing interest in holistic health, there is also a cautious reluctance to abandon conventional medicine, as if having one excludes the other. Fortunately, we do not need to choose one over the other when we know how to select integrated care. This book is designed for people who are seeking greater well-being and for those dealing with

1

disease (meaning anything that gets in the way of living a full life, not being 'at ease') as well as for physicians who are interested in providing 'integrated' care and may not be sure how to do so. This resource guide will educate you about healing options.

The first part of the book is a narrative about my healing experiences. I describe my path and the questions I have asked as well as the answers I have found for myself. I share my path as one example of the struggles inherent in healing. You don't need to have had the same health concerns or life experiences that I've had. I write about universal feelings of powerlessness, despair, and frustration, as well as hope and inspiration, and the desire to know more, find out more, and understand more.

The second part of the book describes healing resources – health centers, hospitals, associations, and educational institutions related to the integration of holistic (alternative) and conventional medicine. With this guide in hand, you won't have to make endless, potentially frustrating calls trying to figure out where to turn. You will be provided with leads to make your search for wellness a fruitful one.

This book doesn't give you easy answers – no one can. This book may or may not save you money, but you will certainly be getting a better value for the money you do spend because you won't be buying services you don't want, need, or understand. You will be more informed about your choices. Of course, the best thing is not to get into a crisis situation. Some resources found in this guide will help you stay well so you'll be less likely to find yourself in crisis.

I do not organize information around disease states and symptoms. We are interrelated systems, and although there may be specific treatments or herbs that work well for treating particular ailments, addressing our health as a *whole* is required to resolve underlying causes of the symptoms.

This book is definitely *not* an argument against conventional medicine. Conventional medicine is undeniably lifesaving and truly miraculous when used appropriately, for medical emergencies, infections, and trauma care. Conventional medicine has been less effective in disease prevention and in dealing with some of today's (environmentally-induced) illnesses, especially chronic ones. For these, conventional medicine alone is not always our best choice, although it is a good idea to get a diagnosis from a medical doctor along with other holistic practitioners. There are many resources available to help in the search for greater well-being and fulfillment. To make the most of what is available, we must educate and listen to ourselves. As people on healing paths continue to join together, we give each other support and encouragement, and each of us in our own way makes the path a little easier for those who travel alongside and behind us.

Our health options are changing. As more people demand integrated care, and physicians and holistic practitioners learn about other fields, our health care system will be forced to change. I hope this guide will help advance necessary changes in medicine, health care, and insurance. Our culture itself is in transition. It is akin to the Wild West out there, and individuals and institutions who have profited by the system are naturally unwilling to let it go. However, the demand for a new system of health care is so high that changes are inevitable.

2

CHAPTER TWO: MY HEALING PATH

The reason I will be telling you so many personal things about myself is so you can see that living a life in balance is challenging, and you're not alone in your struggles. I've tried many different approaches to healing. You don't need to have had the same problems that I've had for this book to be useful for you. I use my path as example, to illustrate struggles that we all go through in different ways. The purpose of this book is to help you – wherever you may be on your own healing path – to become and stay well. In addition to helping you feel great, another purpose of the book is making more options available to health care consumers.

I am writing this book not because I am a health care expert, but because I crossed the boundaries between conventional and non-conventional before it was remotely acceptable. As you will see, I've had my share of personal experiences with conventional and holistic health care, and the thought of ever having to go to a hospital terrified me. The idea for this book came sometime in 1995 because I wanted to know if there were hospitals that provided integrated care, places where patients would be respected and treated holistically. I started doing the research for this book while I was completing my PhD in business, in early 1996. I started the actual writing in January of 1997, and here it is now, many revisions later, in your hands.

Health is much more than the mere absence of disease. Accordingly, healing encompasses more than medical treatment alone. As Jennifer Jacobs, MD, MPH, says so aptly in The Encyclopedia of Alternative Medicine, **"Health is...a state of harmony or balance in the organism. Negative influences in one's life are thought to throw the body out of balance and create illness. Such factors as overwork, family** stress, and excessive anger or grief can affect the mental/ emotional levels of health, while poor eating habits, lack of exercise, exposure to harmful microorganisms, and hereditary tendencies can create illness in the physical sphere." I touch upon subjects that some people might consider outside the realm of health because I consider them to be relevant to the healing process.

As an infant and child I was very sickly. I had asthma attacks requiring emergency visits that I do not remember and after that, oxygen tents at home that I do remember. In elementary school I missed a lot of school because I was sick so much with asthma and allergies. In spite of that, doing well academically was easy for me because I loved learning, but I didn't have energy left for other activities.

Although I have never been critically ill, nor required hospital stays since I was an infant, I grew up chronically ill. As a child my mom carted me from doctor to doctor. Physically I appeared in good working order – too bad for me that I felt miserable and fatigued. There was nothing I could do except take medicine to suppress the symptoms temporarily.

We met doctors who wanted to take out various organs (I don't remember which ones they thought weren't really necessary!), to see what would happen. Fortunately my mom declined their offers. I am not exaggerating when I say that until I was twenty-five I was sick every day. Not in bed sick every day, but I always suffered from a cold, allergies, flu, stomachache, menstrual cramps or occasional asthma attacks. When I complained that I felt sick, my brothers would say, "No offense, Beth, but what's new?".

My family moved from California to Connecticut when I was in kindergarten. In third grade, when I was eight, we moved to Paris, where we lived for five years, until I was thirteen. My asthma attacks disappeared sometime around our move to Paris. Before we moved my mom started learning how to give injections because our doctor wouldn't be coming to our house in the middle of the night anymore to give me the shots himself. As I watched her practicing with apples and oranges I became terrified that she wouldn't give me the shot properly and I would be killed by an air bubble that she hadn't seen. I never needed a shot after that! I still travel with an inhaler even though it's been about twenty years since I've had an asthma attack.

My earliest memory of trying to improve my health is from when we lived in Paris. I was always sick and hated it. I was tired all the time and felt that I was missing all the fun because I was often at home, sick in bed. I remember going on a 'be healthy' kick and waking up early in the morning to run down a closed off side street near our apartment. I would take off my coat and put my school bag down, and run to the end of the block and back, and then breathless, pick up my belongings and go to school. I also tried walking to and from school (about an hour walk) for a short while, but I don't remember any difference in how I felt.

We moved back to Connecticut when I was thirteen. In high school I tried healthy diets, yoga, meditation, eliminating sugar, and so on. I bought a 'how-to meditate in 30 days' book and woke up extra early every morning to do the weird things the book told me to do. Lighting candles, sitting quietly, putting my body in different positions. I tried so hard to do it right. I don't remember feeling anything but a sense of failure. I did not 'get it' and clearly could not do it the right way.

I hated feeling sick all the time and nothing doctors gave me seemed to help me feel better. In high school I told my family doctor that I didn't think I was eating well because I ate about 3 candy bars a day (and not much at meal times). He said that was nothing to worry about. I started visiting holistic health providers who believed in nutrition, and the importance of strengthening the immune system. Responsibility and self-care were required as part of healing. These practitioners would not prescribe medication or surgery to 'cure' the patient. There was no magic pill.

In my late teens I went to a 'no-frills' health spa. In the early eighties spas were not yet in vogue, and they were basically places to lose weight, not places for people to enhance their health. I weighed less than one-hundred pounds and went to the spa for fitness and spiritual renewal, yet most people at the spa, including the staff, assumed I was there to lose weight and convincing them to give me second helpings of food was difficult! The food was healthy and delicious. It was during this spa visit that I met a man in his seventies who gave me his secret for ending constipation. He told me to drink at least eight glasses of water a day, walk briskly daily, and sit on the toilet every morning at the same time to train the body. It works.

In college I wanted to be released from the dormitory food contract because the food was so unhealthy. I needed to get a medical release from a physician, so I went to the student health services and spoke with a doctor. When I told him I believed that white bread and sugar were not as good for you as unrefined products (whole grains and natural sweeteners) he referred me to a psychiatrist to help with my 'eating disorder'. I was struggling against a system which endorsed the medical model of health. Nutrition and lifestyle were not believed to be connected with physical health. It was not commonly believed that our mind, lifestyle, or diet had any connection with illness.

Most of my adult life I have experimented with various 'health' diets in the attempt to feel better. Some of these diets were strict while others were more lenient. I now believe that there is much more to good health than the food we put in our bodies. Enjoying ourselves, enjoying the eating experience, and eating in moderation are probably better for us than the healthiest diet that causes negative feelings of deprivation, resentment, or guilt.

In the effort to make myself healthy, I suffered miserably because I did not do everything I thought I 'should' be doing. My experience has taught me that any practice which instills guilt for not adhering to it rigidly can not be healthy. When we feel guilty for not following a program or practice perfectly rather than feeling proud of what we have done, we are injuring ourselves and using 'shoulds' to beat ourselves up.

It is helpful to be reminded periodically that we are all human. We were not made to be perfect, so requiring perfection from ourselves is futile and in a way disrespectful. We need to acknowledge the good things we have done. If we do not stick to something perfectly, so be it. Forgive, be gentle, and move on. That is probably one of the least recognized tenets of good health: be gentle with yourself. Don't 'should' on yourself!

After college I moved to Massachusetts and worked for a public interest consumer advocacy and environmental lobbying group. I became frustrated with the lack of structure, and what I perceived to be fanaticism and unprofessionalism in the organization, so I quit after about half a year. I spent the rest of the year scooping ice-cream in Northampton for the original creator of 'mix-ins'. I could eat anything I wanted while I worked there and literally made myself sick with ice-cream concoctions. What a way to go! My favorite creation was a chocolate malt with oreos and hot fudge blended in.

In the summer of 1986, I moved to California and worked for a health care consortium in San Francisco and then went to school in Berkeley for a Master's Degree in Public

Health (MPH). I did a six-month internship with Kaiser Permanente in Portland, Oregon as part of the MPH program. While I was living in Berkeley I became familiar with the Macrobiotic diet which is vegetarian and dairy-free, and recommends eating certain foods in prescribed portions. There was a macrobiotic restaurant in nearby Oakland that served wonderful tasting and reasonably priced macrobiotic meals. The restaurant was part of a house with a grocery store. It had a very communal, friendly nature. Volunteers could prepare and serve meals in exchange for a free meal. I volunteered a few times, and those experiences turned out to be among the best cooking classes I ever had. As a former professor of mine said, "more can be caught than taught". By working alongside cooks, I learned more about preparing macrobiotic meals than I learned in cooking classes.

People in the macrobiotic community were very strict about following the diet: precise proportions of grains, beans, certain vegetables, and no dairy or meat. Eating other foods was pretty much taboo. Some people went to such extremes that it became impossible for them to eat out with non-macrobiotic people. They needed to prepare food themselves or have it prepared by others who adhered to macrobiotic requirements. It was supposed to cure all ills. If you didn't feel better, it was your fault for not following the diet strictly enough. Macrobiotic followers have mellowed considerably since then. The macrobiotic diet, generally speaking, is not a bad diet. Many of the recommendations are in line with other nutritional authorities and established guidelines in favor of a mostly vegetarian, low-fat, whole food diet. It was the fanaticism and rigidity that really got to me. I never experienced the health I expected, no matter how strict I was. Later I found that I had food allergies, especially to wheat. I never felt the well-being that I expected from following the macrobiotic diet, in large part because I was eating foods I was allergic to at every meal!

While living in Berkeley I also experimented with homeopathy and acupuncture (these approaches are defined in the Treatment Chapter). I felt slightly better with each practice, but never anywhere near well. I was exhausted, had a cold or flu every day, and constant stomachaches. I continued my search when I moved to Portland. I saw a naturopath and started getting colonics (cleansing of the bowels). Eventually the naturopath referred me to a food allergist and I found out I was sensitive to many foods and chemicals. I began a strict rotation diet where I ate only a single food at each meal, and then did not eat that food again for 4 days, and I did not eat any foods in that food family for 2 days. After a few weeks, I could eat 2 foods at a meal, and so on. I rotated foods for almost a year. I also received injections to lessen the food and chemical sensitivities. I no longer have any concerns with food allergies.

When I graduated with my Master's degree in Public Health in 1989, I moved to Ann Arbor and did consulting projects. My health had once again plateaued. I felt better than before, but not well. I decided to visit a famous allergy specialist in Syracuse, N.Y. My brother, who drove with me from our parents' home in Connecticut and accompanied me for moral support, was shocked at the pains they took to provide an allergy free environment. No dust, no chemicals or scents were permitted on persons or their clothing, and there were air filters all over the place. The hard work of following a rotation diet and avoiding as many chemicals as I could did pay off – now I eat whatever I want without worrying about allergies. This was not the only key to my over all well-being, but it was definitely a very significant improvement.

In 1990 I took a bicycle trip across the U.S. That was truly something I never thought I would be able to do. I only attempted it because a friend who also had tendencies to be sickly and needed to take good care of her health wanted me to go with her, and she promised we would cook healthy meals for ourselves along the way. We did, in fact, manage to eat pretty well on our trek across the U.S. I left the group mid-way because of a pre-arranged trip I had to take in July, but I rejoined them a few days outside of Washington, DC, our destination point, and rode in with the group. With that amazing feat behind me, I started business school at the University of Chicago, where I received both my MBA (1993) and Ph.D. (1996). I went to business school to learn more about the managerial aspects of starting a health center. I specialized in Total Quality Management (TQM), a management philosophy that involves many disciplines in the pursuit of continuous improvement. TQM philosophy is similar to holistic health care philosophy because at the heart of both is the belief in finding and resolving the root causes of an issue rather than exclusively treating symptoms.

I discovered **Ayur-Veda,** a diet/healing system originating in India and made popular in the U.S. by Deepak Chopra, MD, while I was in business school. The philosophy and practices feel very natural to me. Chopra never fails to inspire me. When I read *Perfect Health,* so much resonated with me - it just felt right. When I discovered that people with my mind-body type should avoid cold drinks and foods (because we are by nature already cold, and more cold is imbalancing for us), I got so excited. I was not the only person in the world to order water without ice in restaurants! Recommendations are given regarding food and diet, exercise, and stress reduction for different mind-body types, of which there are 3 (vata, pitta, kapha). People may be a single mind-body type or a combination of two, or in rare cases a combination of all three. There are simple written tests to determine what type you are, although pulse diagnoses by ayur-vedic physicians are more reliable. The Treatment Chapter provides greater explanation about Ayur-Veda.

I see an ayur-vedic physician and participate in *pancha-karma* (a healing program) every year and a half or so and find the visits insightful and inspiring. I understand more about myself and what I need to do to feel better. Every time I see an ayur-vedic physician I add more practices to my regular routines. I don't feel overwhelmed by it, I feel hopeful and inspired. I have done Transcendental **Meditation** and now do Primordial Sound Meditation (an ancient Indian technique revived by Deepak Chopra) regularly. Once I stopped trying to force an outcome, meditation became effortless. When I have thoughts, I just bring my attention back to my mantra without making myself wrong. These meditation practices are 20-30 minute blocks of time where one quiets the mind and the body is relaxed. I used to do it twice every day, and found it deeply restful. I have been out of the habit for a while and am now getting back to it because I have really missed how peaceful and rested I felt when I practiced daily.

While I was in college I discovered a book and meditation tape by **Shakti Gawain**. This was one of my first exposures to creative visualization. Her books and tapes (*especially* her tapes because she has such a soothing voice) guide you into that place in your mind/spirit where you can create and then manifest your desires into physical reality.

I took a course called the **Silva Method** for Mind Control right before my cross-country bike trip. When I was in college I bought a book about the Silva Method which taught the techniques to reach the 'alpha' state, a highly creative and relaxed state. I didn't have much success with the book, but I found the course very powerful. Through self-guided visualization you learn how to heal yourself and others, how to relax, and how to program the brain for specific tasks like sleeping better, remembering what you read, or bringing about specific events. Tuition is a one-time charge, and after you graduate you can take the course again, at any time.

I have participated in programs offered by **Landmark Education Corporation** for the last several years. Their work teaches breakthrough thinking. By learning about the design principles of human beings, one gains the ability to make different choices in daily life. In the Landmark Forum, the foundation course, participants examine and challenge fundamental assumptions about what is possible. Life becomes much more of a choice, and the emphasis is on being in action, not watching life from the sidelines.

I find health spas and retreats to be wonderful places for reconnecting with my self and for rejuvenation. Other activities which I engage in to support my well-being are: an **Artist's Way** circle, using Julia Cameron's book as our guide, **Tai Chi** classes, and **yoga**, which is helping me breathe deeper and be more flexible.

A Holistic Path

I did not choose to be interested in holistic medicine; it chose me. I wanted desperately to feel better and live a more fulfilling life. So, I was willing to try anything that seemed promising. Many 'conventional' beliefs never made sense to me anyway. For example, as a child I remember thinking how bizarre it was that companies would refine a product, like white flour, taking all the nutrients out of it and then add vitamins and minerals back. I did not understand why foods were altered rather than eaten in their natural states. Processing was expensive as well as compromising to the health value of the food. In later years I started to understand how the tastes to which we become accustomed fuel the desire for artificial and convenience foods which are huge and profitable industries in this country.

It also seemed obvious to me that food additives, smoking, and dangerous environmental toxins were major contributors to cancers and other illness. Twenty years ago we heard very little about how the polluted environment, chemical additives, and smoking could contribute to cancer. Instead, large amounts of money were spent on research to reverse rather than prevent diseases. Only later did the hazards of smoking and releasing chemicals into the environment enter into discussions about cancer and other illnesses. Then I began to understand how powerful industrial lobbies could keep certain issues quiet.

I wasn't getting well with regular medicine, and I was open to unconventional alternatives that would help me be healthy. Holistic approaches, which require the participation of the person who is being healed, appealed to me. Being involved in our own care, and taking responsibility for healing is *not to be confused with taking blame for being unwell.* Taking responsibility for your health means that you are willing to inquire into why you are unwell and actively take steps to change it. It does not mean that you wanted to be sick, or you made yourself unwell, or that if you were a better person you would not feel the way you do.

In addition to being sick, you may also feel guilty for being sick! Guilt comes in different forms. There is the self-imposed guilt: what did I do to make myself sick? Where did I fail in being well? What am I doing wrong or not well enough? And there is other-imposed guilt, with other people asking: "How come you are sick again?", "Why don't you take care of yourself better?" And then there is the guilt we make up, being embarrassed to say that we are sick because others may think badly of us.

I heard a very sad story about a woman suffering from cancer who died with a book of affirmations by her side, all the time feeling she had failed by not doing something right. We are *not to blame* for being unwell. I think holistic practitioners in the past may have, at some level, blamed the unwell person for his/her condition. It used to be common to ask questions such as "what did you do to bring this upon yourself?" These questions may be well meaning, but they can have terrible effects on the people who are healing themselves. A more gentle approach is commonly found now, working in partnership to discover what message is being conveyed so that it can be addressed and the person can heal.

Treating the symptom alone does not necessarily resolve the underlying issue, or deeper cause. *Holistic approaches will reach beyond the presenting symptom and look for the underlying issues.* Creating a partnership with your practitioner is the result of approaching the relationship as an equal. You have a right to understand what is going on and to be treated with respect, as a "whole" human being, not as the symptom(s) for which you are being treated.

Although being sick feels bad, it is not necessarily a bad thing. I do not know of anyone who wants to be sick, but there are things to be learned from being sick that we might not have

15

learned without the illness. Symptoms are the body's (or mind/spirit's) way of bringing awareness to something that needs attention. If we do not hear a quiet knock, it may take a full blown catastrophe for us to get the message! Listening for the subtle messages in our lives will lead to a greater sense of well-being and probably better health too. You are not to blame for being sick. You did not do anything wrong. Although there may still be physical manifestations of disease, as you heal in other dimensions and other areas of your life, pain and anxiety may be diminished.

If you believe illness is a message given to us, then deciphering the message can be very helpful to the healing process. For example, I found that being sick was an acceptable excuse for not doing something I didn't want to do anyway. I found that when I stopped using illness as an excuse, even though I really was sick, then I stopped being sick as frequently. For example, I would go to meetings or social engagements when I said I would, even if I felt tired or sick, and then I would feel better when I was there. If I didn't want to go somewhere I would say no instead of saying yes, and then later become ill. The message was to find and use my voice - to speak up for myself rather than letting my illness speak for me. Other important messages that illness brings: slow down, don't live at such a hectic pace, and *pay attention to yourself.*

Holding an unwell person responsible for being sick, like blaming the victim, is the same as 'shoulding' on someone. Saying what a person should have done or should do is not conducive to healing. Illness is often a message, something we can learn from, and we all learn and heal in our own ways. Sometimes healing happens without physical improvements. If a person leaves a dissatisfying job, or a destructive relationship, or tells someone significant to them that they love them, then healing may occur regardless of what is happening in their body. Being healed is a mind/body/emotion state; *it is possible to be healed and be physically unwell,* although that is not what most of us would think of as our ideal state.

Just because something worked for someone else, that doesn't mean it will work for you. An approach or substance may work miracles for your friend while doing absolutely nothing for you. Your body chemistry is different than your friend's, so the same therapy may have different effects. Trying to fix other people because something works well for you isn't a good idea. It is annoying when people do it to me, and I am beginning to realize the futility of doing it to other people. I am an intelligent person and I appreciate hearing about other people's experiences (most of the time), but I do not always want to be told what to do or why I am sick.

I continuously remind myself that my path toward well-being is legitimate, that my way is the right way for me, in fact the only way for me. I consider doing activities which keep me well to be part of my 'work'. Seeking wellness could be part of everyone's 'work', if that is what they choose. Taking the time to care for yourself (massage, yoga, meditation, eating well, blocks of time for relaxing) can be thought of as selfish, yet if you aren't well, how can you accomplish other goals or take care of other people?

Following your own path is a difficult thing, and it requires courage and time. It can be hard to follow your dream because of skepticism, cynicism, time constraints and attacks from the outside world and from your own 'censor'. Your censor is that part of you that tells you it is not okay to think or say something that might be risky. It is easier to do what society expects.

It is important to put time in your schedule for yourself. Healing really can be a component of any lifestyle, once you make a commitment to it, even if it's only one 'little thing' at a time. Healing is a process, not an end point. There is not just one healing path, or a single legitimate way. There are many roads to Rome, as the saying goes, and many ways to find healing for yourself. *Finding your own purpose and following it* is a key to healing. It helps to know that what works for you might (and in fact is likely to) be different from what others have found for themselves.

17

Finding your soul's work, your life's purpose, is a fundamental part of healing. There are many ways to discover your self, your purpose, and your ways of healing. It is easy to say that it does not matter whether people agree with you or endorse what you are doing, but living with real or perceived disagreement may be a challenge to self worth and esteem. Meeting this challenge is part of gaining inner strength and following our own path. This is not to say that a traditional job is bad for your health. However, if your work compels you to neglect your *self* then something needs to change if you are to maximize well-being: either the job, or how your life is structured so that time for healing, and the commitment to healing, can co-exist with your job.

All human beings have the desire to express themselves, be understood, and contribute to others' lives. To heal ourselves, and in so doing heal our planet, we each need to explore and find what is right for us (and this will change at different times). Although we live in a culture which looks outside ourselves to experts, no one can tell someone else what is right for him or her. Healing requires being comfortable listening to our inner wisdom. All of us can use guides, but guides are meant to be used as partners in learning, healing, and self-exploration; guides are not the definitive authority. Self-expression and self-exploration are integral parts of knowing yourself and this helps the healing process, but it is not always enough. They are only steps on the path, not the whole path.

As a society we are used to quick fixes. This applies to our health care too. We have come to expect an authority, usually our medical doctor, to know what is ailing us and to cure the problem without much effort on our part. Holistic health takes another approach. *We are the authority, we are responsible for our healing.* We seek guidance from people with expert knowledge that may help us, but we are in charge. Medical doctors do not know everything; they are artists like all other healers, and can only guide us. We are responsible for listening to our bodies and asking questions about our choices.

18

Our old model of healing placed the physician in the expert position. He knew best, and we did not question anything or ask for more information. We did not need to understand, we needed only to follow his directions. Holistic practitioners, including physicians, foster partnerships with the person seeking healing. They serve as facilitators, using their knowledge and expertise to aid the healing person in tapping into their own inner wisdom and healing themselves. Our life is a path of self-discovery: finding ways of fulfilling our purpose and helping others. Healing involves bringing our life into alignment, so we are consistent about what we say and what we do. When you honor your word for all the little things (keeping promises to yourself and to others), then it becomes more automatic to believe that you will do what you proclaim in terms of larger goals as well.

Pleasing people can interfere with the healing process if you are neglecting your own needs. People who live their lives only to please others are not always happy or well. Sacrificing yourself for the sake of sacrifice does not honor you as a person, and is not conducive to healing. Avoiding conflict (suppressing issues and feelings) doesn't pay! It will come out one way or another, and often in illness or disease. When we learn to come from a place of love and forgiveness, for ourselves as well as for others, then we will find ourselves saying what needs to be said in compassionate ways. Of course, remember, we are still human and will never say everything perfectly all the time. When you mess up, clean up the mess and forgive yourself. When someone else messes up, forgive them. It is healthier for you!

Suppressing our shadow selves (our dark sides that we don't want to acknowledge as part of us) is related to pleasing people. We all have parts of ourselves that we are not eager for other people to see. When these parts are denied, they won't stay repressed forever. At some point, most likely when you least expect it, you will experience some kind of blow up, or perhaps an illness will emerge as a result of stifling your self expression. There are many different ways of safely expressing your 'shadow' self, from the creative arts (see Julia Cameron's books, *The Artist's Way* and *The Vein of Gold*), to self-discovery workshops, to transformational courses, to a variety of healing approaches.

We tend to have such high expectations of ourselves. I have heard people say that they are a disappointment to God or are not doing enough with their lives, or feel overwhelmed with all they could or should be doing. We often limit ourselves by using age, time constraints, low confidence, or creative sabotaging techniques. Becoming aware of our creative strategies for sabotage is an important step in learning how to overcome them, and being unstoppable in reaching our dreams. This applies to healing ourselves as well. We sabotage ourselves in many different ways, such as surrounding ourselves with people who reinforce our negative and limiting beliefs, or by filling our days with low priority (but perhaps 'urgent') tasks. It is not intentional and does not make us bad or wrong. Our task is to become well, being gentle with ourselves and understanding the lessons our body/spirit is telling us. With heightened awareness, messages that otherwise might not have been noticed until they develop into a full blown health crisis are more likely to be detected and heeded at earlier stages.

I believe in being straightforward about what you want and what you feel. I am in favor of being flexible and reaching win-win solutions, but there is slim possibility for optimal agreement if people are not saying what they really want (especially if they are just trying to be nice and please other people). When we follow paths that are not our own, that is, do things to please someone else when it goes against what we believe, then things have a higher probability of not working out.

Sometimes in conversations where other people try to fix me, I feel like I am bad or wrong for feeling the way I do, and that it's my fault I do not feel well. I must remind myself, this is my path. Right or wrong do not apply. I will do what I do, and I will get the results I get. That is what it means to stay on your path. It is your path, and no one knows it like you do! Do what you need to do, while still taking in information and guidance from whatever sources you find useful. We all need to find out for ourselves what works, and not push what has worked for us on others, much as we want to help other people.

Sometimes people need to take time off simply to decompress. Most people's first reaction to this is that taking time off is not financially possible for them. This may be true, but don't dismiss the possibility of taking time off without exploring all options. After all, think of how much it would cost if you were seriously ill and required hospitalization. Insurance is unlikely to cover all your expenses, and you would still have to pay something. Wouldn't that money be better spent in the effort to keep you well? Are there people in your life who can pitch in for you (baby-sit the kids if that's needed, let you borrow their home if they're away so you can have a mini-retreat)?

One friend told me about someone who simply went to her boss, explained her need to take a month off to "decompress", and was shocked when her boss said okay. According to her boss, it would have taken at least a month to replace her, so she considered it a "mental health sabbatical." The boss is now considering doing the same thing herself!

If not working is an option for you, you may have to contend with other people's opinions about what you should be doing if you stay unemployed for 'too long'. Even if we have people close to us who are supportive, it can be difficult to take the time to care for ourselves because of what we think others might be thinking, or because of the effects on our self-esteem. In our society, taking time off from 'earning money' and putting one's attention fully on one's own well-being is not validated. We may believe that, in addition to surviving, we must be working for money to have self-esteem, and be worthy in the eyes of others.

Unfortunately, many of us can talk more freely about difficulties than we can about good fortune. We do not want to engender potential envy. It is not acceptable to talk too much about how well things are going; we might put people off who think we are boasting, or trying to make them feel bad. It is more acceptable to commiserate about hardships than it is to say how great life is. When people talk about good fortune they are apt to tone it down by saying, don't worry, I have had plenty of troubles in the past, or I'm sure it is just temporary. People seem to be embarrassed to speak openly about how wonderful their life is. We commonly bond by sharing our troubles and pain. My point is only that we live in a culture that supports the sharing of pain more than pleasure. Since words are so powerful, I find complaining to be an energy zapper. Focusing on the negative seems to bring on more negatives.

Our society is beginning to acknowledge that you do not have to do something you hate in order to survive. More books and workshops are becoming available on the subject of finding work you love and making a living doing it. Yet, 'following your bliss' can be a difficult path. One reason people are often discouraged from doing what they love is the fear that they will not be able to support themselves. It is risky to follow one's inner vision, and it is easy to see why well meaning friends and family would caution us not to be foolish. Paradoxically, it is this very aversion to risk taking, meant to protect us, which prevents the full expression of self and is damaging to our soul. We need to heed our vision, and then take the appropriate actions to bring our dreams into existence. Knowing your path is one thing; following it is a different matter.

Following **my holistic path** started as a struggle against being sick and tired. I saw doctors, specialists, and alternative healers; participated in seminars and workshops; went to spas and health clinics; and read numerous books and articles about wellness. I am a searcher by nature and am driven to explore new experiences: Practitioner after practitioner, book after book, health diet after health diet, meditation after meditation, exercise program after program. Working hard in itself does not do the trick. Being gentle with yourself (and still disciplined) is far more effective. Do the best you can, strive to do better, and acknowledge yourself for all that you are doing.

Constituting Beliefs and Practices

I think I was born 'grown up'. I see pictures of myself at four and five, and already I am an efficient, serious person. My second grade report card says that I am a real little lady. My dad used to refer to me as Ms. Put Together. I was raised with the belief that I could do anything. I am fortunate to have had an upbringing that infused me with confidence and a feeling that I am competent, smart, likable and lovable. Still, there are many things I have had to work out, such as expressing my anger appropriately instead of suppressing it. (One of the Golden Rules in my family is 'Make People Happy.') I've gotten much better at straight talk, telling someone truthfully what there is to say instead of avoiding what is uncomfortable.

Even if we are fortunate enough to have had picture perfect childhoods, just by being human we all have fears, hurts, and shame within us. Delving into them and resolving them as adults is a very worthwhile endeavor. It has very much to do with our healing, quality of life and our relationships. It takes a great deal of courage to look closely inside ourselves and how we work. What we find is not always pretty! Remember when you see something about yourself that you don't like, that does not make you a bad person – be gentle with yourself.

Another key to happiness and well-being is not making others wrong. 'Make wrong' is in our make up, and what we get from being right is BEING RIGHT! We do not get love, intimacy or affinity with people. On the contrary, being right actively detracts from all that. *Try giving up being right. It is hard to do, but the rewards are great.* Loving is better for your health. Sometimes when I am arguing with someone, I just love *being right,* and being right about whatever we are talking about becomes more important than the relationship itself. When that is happening, there is no room for loving, or

23

even liking that person. When I become aware of this situation and choose to stop being attached to being right, then there is fertile ground which moments before had been stark and fallow. It's a good feeling.

I am a very organized person, good at planning and scheduling. I live by my day planner. Everything I need to know is in there. Everyday I efficiently check off tasks accomplished and put a little arrow on those that have not been completed, and move them to another day. Sometimes I move tasks for weeks. But they always get done (or they fall off the list and drive me crazy until they are completed or discarded). The other side of this is that I am a little – what's the right word – compulsive. Things need to be done efficiently. I need to squeeze something out of every minute, even if I make myself sick or anxious in the process. Being aware that I have a tendency to do this has helped me to slow down and allow things to happen rather than forcing outcomes all the time.

Like most people, I want people to like me, and deep down I think that if I disagree with someone about something I will not be liked. This is a little paradoxical because all my life I have been a pioneer. Here I was, this 'together', bright young woman, yet a proponent of *unconventional* practices. I believed and spoke openly about *possibility*. I was doing what I loved with my life, which included not working in a traditional career. I don't believe that life has to be a struggle, nor do I believe that we must suffer. Lots of people do not think I am doing life 'right'. It is too easy. While everything is not always 'nice' or 'comfortable', we don't have to be victims of circumstances. Stuff happens – how we deal with it is up to us.

Being a pioneer sometimes meant being a loner. I wanted the support of others, and I wanted to be reassured that I was doing the right thing, or at least a valued thing. I was a vegetarian in the early 1980s, when most people thought that only weirdos were vegetarians. Now being a vegetarian is acceptable. People are more familiar with vegetarianism, and the media coverage is generally favorable. This is quite a change from 15 years ago.

I believe in some cosmic force, call it God or supreme being or cosmic will. When an intention is stated clearly, the universe will provide for the manifestation of it as long as it is not harmful to another. We may not always be aware of our intent being met, so the more specific you are, the better. I've been taught that bad intentions will backfire – if you were to wish ill on someone, you could count on the same coming to you. Personally, I know I feel better when I have compassion for someone instead of holding them as a supreme jerk.

My belief in the good of the universe has allowed me to feel protected and cared for. I have the firm belief that I can do whatever I am meant to do and everything will always turn out well. So, I choose differently from other people and I stick with it. It takes courage, but I also do not feel like I have much choice. I have to do what I do because that is who I am. This is where your spiritual beliefs come into play. Many people find that their spiritual/religious beliefs help them cope better with their health and life circumstances. I find that spiritual beliefs help me find peace and joy, which I think are instrumental to healing.

I used to get turned off when people talked about God. It does not bother me anymore, I just substitute my own words: universe, higher power, higher self, cosmic will. I believe there is a cosmic force at work, guiding and coordinating everything. Synchronicity, or serendipity, is always at work whether we notice it or not. There are times in my life when I am more aware of synchronicity than others. Above all, when I let go, and let the universe take care of me, everything goes smoothly, effortlessly, and easily. When I try to force an outcome I get into trouble. I still work hard when I let go, I just release control, and when I do that I stop worrying. Sometimes I see lessons for myself in situations and sometimes I don't.

I need a lot of time alone. Being in social situations or at school or work can sometimes be exhausting. I used to strongly dislike being in situations that I could not control. I have always been more comfortable being at home than anywhere else. In that respect I am a little bit of a homebody, even though I have fun with people and at parties. In my younger days I was reluctant to go to parties or on field trips if I could not leave when I wanted to. I was always afraid I would get sick. When I travel, which I love doing, I am still worried I will get sick (and require medical attention or just feel miserable) on my trip. I rarely get sick anymore, but the worry is still very much with me.

It's hard to pinpoint exactly how I moved from being a sick person who had occasional days of relative good health, to being a healthy person who occasionally gets sick. It started after college when I found a wonderful, healing practitioner who understood my problems. I don't remember what supplements he gave me, but I started feeling more energetic. It was probably a combination of the supplements, change of lifestyle to accommodate more time for resting and light exercise, and a more relaxed state of mind. The next leap came when, at the age of 25, I found out I had food allergies and chemical sensitivities.

For the next five or six years I worked mostly with diet, exercise, and visualization. The next major jump in healthiness came when I learned Transcendental Meditation and began following Ayur-Vedic recommendations. In 1995, I began taking courses at Landmark Education Corporation where I dealt with some of the spiritual/emotional components of health and vitality. Now I am a well person.

One of the most important ingredients to well-being is joy. Expressing love and compassion, toward yourself and others, and appreciating the gift that your condition or situation brings you are wonderful healers. I know it might sound hard or impossible to believe that something good could come from something bad. What are some things you can do when you are not feeling joy and you would like to? Make a list of things that make you happy. Pull out the list when you want to feel joy, and do something on it. My list includes picking Angelic Messenger Cards which are beautiful cards with an accompanying book giving the meanings for each card (Angelic Messenger Cards, "A Divination System for Spiritual Self-Discovery" by Meredith L. Young-Sowers are produced by Stillpoint Publishing and cost $29.95); listening to music that makes me feel good (either happy, upbeat tunes or meditative nature music); calling a friend who I can laugh with; reading a book; or listening to a story or lecturer (like Deepak Chopra or Carolyn Myss) on tape. Regular practices like meditating, walking, volunteering and helping others, and reminding myself of the abundance of the universe are very useful too.

Healing requires being gentle and forgiving, with yourself and others. A sense of humor also can do much to relieve the significance, and hence the stress, of problems in our lives. Humor and exercise are two important facets of wellness. Along with humor, exercise, and being gentle and forgiving, having friends and being a friend are paramount. Friends are the greatest blessing and wealth in my life. Having a large network of friends and colleagues enables me to find whatever resources I need easily. Friends are facilitators to healing: research has shown that people with support networks are in better health than those without (See "Social Support: How Friends, Family, and Groups can help," by David Spiegel, MD, in *MindBody Medicine*, listed in Section I: Publications).

Love and forgiveness, besides being nice things, actually have tremendous impacts on our health and healing. So, the next time you are angry with someone, try forgiving them so you feel better! Holding on to anger allows it to live on in our bodies. Repressing our feelings will show up in physical manifestations. Taking care of ourselves in a gentle, compassionate, nonjudgmental way and being the same way with others feels good and is good for us. It is not as easy to do as to talk about, and I have found books, workshops, and talking with friends essential to living this way. In a similar vein, I have heard people talk about the importance of cooking with love in your heart because that imparts energy to the food and those who consume it. *Healing With Love*, by Leonard Laskow, MD, provides references to research about the transfer of energy.

You might be someone who is seeking to make things better (continuous improvement). You might like changes. However, change is scary to many people because of the uncertainty ('the only person who likes change is a baby with a dirty diaper'). Resisting change is normal. Our natural state often seems to be to prefer suffering over change because change is an unknown. At least we know what we have now, whereas the future is unknown. That is why we often do things to sabotage ourselves, even though we say we want change. Deep down, we know it is scary and some powerful part of us wants things just the way they are, thank you very much. *Changing anything in our lives can (and probably will) be met with resistance – by our bodies, by people in our lives, or by circumstances. Know this and push forward anyway.*

The bottom line to creating and following your path to healing is to explore your options with an open mind and a healthy skepticism. Ask yourself how does this fit for me? Try it on, and if it does not feel right, leave it. There is abundance in the universe. It is okay to leave something if it does not feel right for you. Never take on a practice or work with a practitioner if you feel it might be harmful to you or if you have misgivings, even if you do not know why. If you are afraid of something new or uncertain, it is okay to try it anyway; if you are feeling something else, trust your intuition. You are the one who pays the money, takes the medicine (so to speak), and experiences the effects.

Sensuality

What is sensuality doing in this healing resource guidebook? Sensuality and sexuality are essential components of healing. They are very integral parts of our identity and self-expression, and connected to our energy flow. When there are blockages in this area, it can affect other parts of our system and life. We are, after all, holistic beings, and all our parts are interconnected. Sensuality can also be challenging to deal with because of all the social taboos surrounding the subject. I have found that my personal experiences with being female are not unique. I am beginning to accept that I have had mixed feelings about being female. I love being a woman and all the privileges afforded to me because of that, and I also resist being female in some ways. I have always been a feminist, believing that women are complete human beings and deserve the same opportunities and respect as men. But women and men are different, and our challenge is accepting and appreciating these differences without having one sex be greater or more important than the other.

The 'male' way of doing things is often considered better in our society. I wanted to be with the guys, act like one of the guys. From what I saw, being a guy meant being a clearer thinker, a more logical and reasonable person. A linear thinker. That was how I saw my father and other men. My mom seemed like a poor reasoner, very inconsistent and illogical. Now I can see that my mom thinks in a different way that is no less valid or useful, but is not always validated in our (male dominated) world. Linear, logical thinking is more valued than creative thinking. In fact, creative thinking is rarely taught – and is even discouraged – within our school systems that place a heavy emphasis on memorizing 'the right answer'. Jobs traditionally held by men pay better than jobs traditionally held by women, and for reasons other than simple supply and demand.

Women used to have to really prove themselves. In order to be heard and make headway, women had to be forceful and sometimes not behave 'nicely'. We almost had to be militant, and sometimes appear distinctly unfeminine, to make breakthroughs. Because of the hard work that was done by early feminists we can now afford to take a softer stance and a more gentle, individualized approach. Today it is not shocking for women to be athletic or have jobs that used to be occupied exclusively by men. It is acceptable – even expected – for women to work outside the home. And it is not shocking, although unfortunately it is not yet the norm, for women to hold important positions in business and government and other organizations.

I've been told by several psychics that I've been reluctant to own my body (they never said anything about a female body in particular), and I had felt that to be true. I have experienced my body as a burden and a hindrance rather than the temple which houses my soul. I was always sick; my spirit was racing ahead and it was a drag to have this body holding me back. My enthusiasm was boundless, but my physical energy was low. I would push ahead, neglecting to take care of my body. I wouldn't eat well (when I did remember to eat, my diet consisted mostly of sweets, especially chocolate), I was a light sleeper, and I would just work until I dropped. Taking care of my physical well-being always took lower priority than mental tasks. I still have a tendency to work instead of eating properly, exercising, walking, or resting. Excellent advice I was once given is to *work until I am tired, not until I am done because my work is never finished.* Giving myself permission to do this has actually helped me to slow down, which ends up increasing my productivity, not to mention being better for my health!

The reluctance to take care of my physical body combined with being in a female body is reflected in my impatience for feminine practices such as taking the time to do my hair, put make up on, take make up off, wax my legs, and all the other female (bodily) things that need to be done according to our societal rules. I thought it was my feminist beliefs that made me reluctant to wear make up or pretty clothes. Men didn't fuss, why should we? And what difference did it make anyway? I wanted to be taken on my own terms, for who I was, not for how pretty I looked. Yet, my apparent reluctance to do feminine things was perhaps more than a feminist stance. Perhaps I was actually at some level rebelling against being in a body, and a female one at that, as psychics have suggested.

Sex used to be complicated and not entirely enjoyable.

Part of my 'healing', or recovery, or awakening of my creative spirit, involved owning my sensuality. Enjoying sex. Taking care of my body. Wearing warm, comfortable, and good looking clothes. Expressing myself, and since I am in a female body, enjoying the expression of my femaleness. I am healing my sensuality by having fun with aromatherapy and color therapy, and by taking time for myself, slowing down and doing things for my own enjoyment.

I have taken several courses about sensuality and intimacy. In one course, *Basic Sensuality*, I reframed my views about sensuality and sexuality and learned facts about female and male sexuality that I had never known. I didn't know that all women have heat cycles and that women have a lot of creative energy when they are in heat. Men don't have heat cycles but are strongly affected by women in heat. I learned that men don't need to ejaculate to have a complete and satisfactory sexual experience. That was a surprise to me, and to the men who take the course and find it to be true. I left the course having access to more fulfilling sensual experiences, knowing how to have my needs met, and the promise of having my partner really love giving me what I want. Sensuality is one more route to accessing our own inner wisdom, to understanding ourselves.

This section about relationships is included because relationships are something we all have to deal with. They will have an effect on our healing process, even if only an indirect one. Relationships serve as valuable learning experiences too because when we are in relationships, we have the opportunity to learn about ourselves in ways that we could not on our own. Our partners provide huge growth opportunities. Relationships, particularly male/female, have a bearing upon our well-being because they are potential sources of stress and of pleasure. The male/female relationship presents so many mysteries, and so much energy is spent trying to understand what's going on and how to make it better. There are endless courses and books on this subject. A course I have found particularly illuminating is *Celebrating Men, Satisfying Women:*

A Romantic Alternative for Women in the'90s (310/839-4223). It is a one day course for women, leaving participants with a renewed appreciation for men. In the course I saw that I was comparing men not to other men, or even other women, but to an *ideal* woman. I found out that I sometimes didn't see men as men, but as dysfunctional women! No *woman* would *ever* do or say *that!* Species are designed for survival, and men have done a pretty good job and I hadn't appreciated them for who they are and what they do. I find it much easier to be with men and their differences now that I've taken this course.

Dreaming about my perfect partner, my prince charming, my soul mate, began as early as kindergarten for me. As I grew older my fantasy man and relationship evolved – I could describe him and knew everything about him! I lived in a fantasy world. Real life was starkly different. When boys liked me in elementary school I was terrified. The first time I got a love note, in 4th grade, I got nauseous and had to go home. I was afraid to go to school the next day. However, I was lucky – the playboy who had sent me the note had already moved on to his next crush.

Although I always wanted that perfect, understanding boyfriend, I did not date until high school and did not have a boyfriend until my sophomore year in college. When I look back over the years I can see that I really did go out with a lot of guys, and a lot of guys liked me, but I didn't see that at the time. I felt like an ugly duckling. I didn't wear make-up, I was vocal about my feminist views, and I was (and still am) very honest and straightforward. I do not believe in playing games. I also avoided confrontation, and did not want to hurt anyone's feelings, so I didn't know how to tell a guy that I didn't want to see him again. I decided it would be easier to not go out with anyone in the first place. I had a lot of crushes on men and fantasized about relationships with them. Fantasy relationships do not disappoint you, and there is always something to look forward to – he might notice you someday and then you would have a fantastic romantic relationship.

In college I went out with some guys I had crushes on, and then I fell in love. We dated exclusively for a year and a half. I was a little sickly almost all the time. I didn't have much energy left after studying and coping with the emotional demands of the relationship. We had several big fights, broke up periodically and made up again passionately. I loved the way he looked, I loved the way he was in love with me, we had fun, and we laughed. My first love. Our final break up was traumatic and it took about three years for me to recover. We broke up during the summer of 1984.

For the next few years I fantasized romances, dated a little, and mostly pined. My health, however, was getting steadily better. I wonder if all the time alone, without the obligations of a relationship, helped me take care of myself. In 1988 I wrote a letter to my college romance, forgiving him and acknowledging him for all he had meant to me. I did not mail the letter. And that was it. I was finally recovered and ready to move on. We did end up speaking not long after that, when he called me out of the blue, and we were able to complete our relationship. I have not heard from him, or of him, since.

As I've become more accepting of my whole self, including my femininity, I have moved from fantasy romance to real relationships, with their very real challenges and rewards. I find I need a lot of time alone which can be challenging to relationships. I sometimes consider myself 'high maintenance' in the sense that I know what I want and expect to be treated well, and know that I'm worth it! Other people have told me that those qualities make me low maintenance, so I guess it all depends on one's perspective. I enjoy being a very independent person, and I look forward to blending my independence with interdependencies in future romantic relationships.

3

Chapter Three: Your Healing Path

How do you find what you need to increase your sense of well-being? You can begin by educating yourself about your diagnosis and exploring your options. Put your own team of teachers/practitioners together who will support you in your healing process. This healing resource guide is designed to help you in finding practitioners for your team, information about various healing approaches, and places to go for support in healing. We'll begin with some basic definitions.

Alternative therapies are those not yet adopted by the mainstream, that is by conventional, or western, medicine. Any approach to solving health problems that are different from those used by conventional practitioners may be considered alternative. **Mind-body medicine** acknowledges the link between mental and physical realms, and addresses the effect that stress has on health. **Complementary** practices are those which complement rather than replace conventional medical practice. Conventional medical practice is viewed as central, and other practices as optional add-ons. **Holistic** health refers to the way care is provided, caring for the whole person rather than treating isolated symptoms. Although holistic health approaches are technically inclusive of both conventional and non-conventional approaches, in common usage holistic usually refers to alternative, non-conventional approaches.

Holistic embodies a 'whole picture' view of the individual: physical, mental, emotional, and spiritual. Holistic also implies comprehensive, including a variety of healing practices. Although the term holistic may include conventional practices, in the context of this book the term holistic will refer to non-conventional (alternative) practices. **Conventional** and allopathic are used interchangeably to refer to standard (U.S.) medical practices.

Holistic is often used interchangeably with words like complementary, alternative, unconventional and mind-body medicine. Some people like the terms complementary or supplementary, but these terms still regard conventional medicine as the core and everything else as subservient and lesser. I find the term **complementary** confusing. Complementing what? The terms **alternative** and **non-conventional** don't actually describe the disciplines or practices. They tell us only that they are not yet conventional. If a complementary, alternative, or non-conventional practice were to become widespread, it still could not be called allopathic or conventional because of the fundamental differences in approach. Holistic is the only really descriptive term - it isn't defined by what it is not as the other terms tend to be. Other terms do *not* convey the notion that health and well-being are multi-faceted and diverse approaches are needed, and that *treating the symptoms does not resolve the cause(s)*.

Holistic approaches vary tremendously, but all focus on empowering the individual to accept responsibility for healing, and emphasize sound nutrition as a core requirement of health. They all recommend a balanced lifestyle, adequate and appropriate exercise, rest, sleep, and emotional tranquillity as the basis for good health and they treat the whole individual rather than symptoms. **Holistic health care** has been defined as a philosophy of medical care which emphasizes personal responsibility and fosters a cooperative relationship among all persons involved (The American Holistic Medical Association). According to Health Care Futures, holistic approaches generally encompass the following principles:

1. The body has a natural ability to heal itself and to remain stable.
2. The human being is a blend of body, mind and spirit and all or any of these factors may cause or contribute to a health problem.
3. Environmental and social conditions are as important as a person's physical and psychological make-up and may have an equally important impact on their health.

4. Treating symptoms masks the real problem. Root causes must be discovered for healing to occur.
5. Each person is an individual and must be treated as such with individualized treatment programs.
6. Healing progresses better, quicker and more thoroughly if every person takes an active role in their healing and responsibility for their health.
7. Good health is a state of emotional, mental, spiritual and physical 'balance.'
8. There is a natural healing force in the universe. The Chinese call this qi or chi (pronounced chee), the Japanese Ki, and in India it is prana. In the West, it is called the life force or 'natural healing force'. It it the alternative health practitioners job to activate chi in the person or help the person activate it in himself.

Integrated care refers to health care delivered 'holistically', accessing both alternative and conventional practices. Conventional and non-conventional therapies are provided together, accessing whatever is in the best interest of the patient. A range of healing practices and programs are available to the patient, supporting his/her well-being, without rejecting the benefits of conventional medicine. All aspects of a person are addressed: the physical, mental, emotional, and spiritual.

Holistic approaches are not a rejection of modern (conventional) medicine. In cases where standard medical care does offer viable treatments, holistic practices make treatments more comfortable and effective because they offer ways for patients to deal constructively with their symptoms. Holistic, comprehensive health care should be the first resort for non-urgent conditions. Holistic health practices are gaining attention, not necessarily as alternatives to conventional medicine, but also as complementary and supplementary practices. There is widespread frustration with a medical care system that is expensive, often invasive, and sometimes ineffective. As a result, alternative, holistic, complementary health practices are gaining favor. *This book is part of a movement toward health care which incorporates the best of modern medicine and the best of a variety of holistic disciplines in which the individual assumes primary responsibility for his/her own care.*

Benefits of Integrated Care

Sixty to ninety percent of physician visits are in the mind-body (stress related) realm. Herbert Benson, MD has proven that for "the most common conditions that prompt people to seek medical care – including insomnia, hypertension and pain – meditation, prayer or mind-body relaxation techniques can provide as much symptom relief as drugs or any other treatment modern medicine has to offer". Benson estimates that over 75% of all doctor visits are for mind-body related illnesses (SELF Magazine's Special Health Issue: The New American Medicine, Nov. 1996). Lifestyle behaviors, enhancing immune systems, and prevention have major impacts on our current causes of pre-mature death.

Illness and disease (anything less than optimal health), are caused largely by lifestyle factors and can often be prevented and treated with lifestyle changes: eating well, exercising properly, managing stress. Chronic conditions are less likely to be 'cured' with surgery or drugs; holistic therapies (including lifestyle changes) are often more effective.

Back problems, anxiety, headache, insomnia, depression, arthritis, high blood pressure, digestive problems, and allergies are some of the conditions for which people seek alternative care, presumably because they are not having success with conventional medical treatments. The Centers for Disease Control point out that lifestyle modification prevents many cases of heart disease, cancer, cerebrovascular disease and atherosclerosis (hardening of the arteries). Therapies which address lifestyle factors and support changes will make a great difference in our nation's overall health status.

The current medical model usually focuses on interventions targeted at one symptom at a time rather than addressing the root causes of disease and treating the patient as a whole person. People are turning to alternative, or holistic, medicine in large numbers, largely out of frustration with conventional medicine, even when their insurance won't cover treatment. The market for holistic/alternative medicine was recently estimated to be a $14-billion market, growing 30% annually (Crain's Chicago Business, January 27, 1997). A study published in the New England Journal of Medicine (January 28, 1993) estimated that in 1990 Americans made 425 million visits to providers of unconventional medicine, spending approximately $13.7 billion.

Examples of holistic therapies include: acupuncture, massage, nutritional philosophies, healing touch, and homeopathy. James Gordon, MD, in *Manifesto for a New Medicine*, talks about a **new medicine** that "combines conventional and alternative therapies, authoritative treatment with respectful care...appreciates the great value of surgery and drugs but sees them as last resorts, not first choices...understands that each one of us is unique, a whole person – biological, psychological, spiritual – in a total social and ecological environment...This new medicine is as concerned with enhancing wellness as it is with treating illness".

Leading personalities in the holistic field support the blending of holistic and conventional medicine. Andrew Weil, MD says, "Mainstream medicine is definitely the way to go for serious injuries. But let's say I developed chronic pain as a result of [an] accident. Beyond narcotics, mainstream medicine doesn't have much to offer. But several complementary therapies can help. I might try chiropractic, acupuncture, yoga, or massage therapy." And Deepak Chopra, MD says, "I'm not at all opposed to medical technology. But technological medicine undervalues the connection between the mind and body. That's where the alternative therapies excel." Joseph Pizzorno, naturopathic doctor and president of Bastyr University states: "Natural medicines may take a little longer to work, but they're less expensive, have fewer side effects, and don't contribute to the terrible problem we now have with antibiotic-resistant bacteria, a problem caused largely by overuse of pharmaceuticals." (San Francisco Focus, March 1997)

Conventional medicine itself has been undergoing a dramatic shift. The influences that stress, beliefs, attitude, and nutrition have on the physical body is no longer denied. The shift toward the 'new medicine' has actually been going on, slowly, for a while. There are several reasons why the shift toward a new medicine is occurring.

First of all, consumers are demanding integrated care. Lack of compassion and choices in conventional medical treatments, especially since the advent of HMOs, are common complaints. Many of the diseases that plague us are *not* best treated with drugs and surgery. Conventional medicine has failed people with chronic conditions, particularly chronic pain. A chronic condition can be defined as a disease or impairment that is not episodic or acute. Chronic illnesses such as arthritis, asthma, cancer, heart disease, multiple sclerosis, Alzheimer's, Parkinson's, and diabetes tend to be less responsive to conventional remedies. *It has been estimated that almost 100 million people had chronic conditions in 1995* (JAMA Nov. 13, 1996).

Modern medicine is undeniably important, and essential, but there are many things it does not adequately address, such as how to support our innate healing processes. Allopathic medicine, with its arsenal of miracle medicines and surgeries, is not the most appropriate response for conditions which are best addressed with lifestyle changes. Emergency care is wonderful for emergencies, but not so wonderful for conditions that need to be treated with less drastic interventions, in a supportive, ongoing manner. Lifestyle changes, prevention and holistic therapies are better than conventional interventions (such as chemotherapy and surgery) for lifestyle related illnesses.

Physicians benefit from integrated care because they have more options to offer patients. Physicians can be frustrated and discouraged when nothing they do for a patient works. Having alternatives, especially less costly, less drastic ones, is better for the physician, the patient, and the patient's family.

On a societal level, our system of health care poses a huge problem: it is extremely expensive to pay for costly hospitalization, medical visits, surgery and drugs. Holistic therapies are, in general, far less costly, and many believe far more cost-effective. If the first resort is self-care and prevention, and low cost holistic therapies instead of physician visits and expensive tests, then the cost of care goes down. Primary care, which is what holistic care consists of, is less costly than surgery, drugs, and emergency room visits.

Choosing the Right Treatments and Practitioner

There are, of course, caveats concerning holistic care. We want alternatives that work, or at least do no harm. People who are ill are vulnerable to poor treatment from *both* conventional and alternative practitioners. Any medical doctor can call himself a 'holistic' medical doctor, even if his only qualification is having read one book. Personal empowerment and listening to our own intuition closely are important parts of the healing process.

The benefits of alternative therapies are beginning to fall under close scrutiny. The Office of Alternative Medicine (OAM) was formed in 1992 as part of the National Institutes of Health. They are funding research into the efficacy of selected alternative therapies. Holistic therapies promise to be effective, less costly than conventional medicine, and more empowering for the individual.

There are many good practitioners and many bad practitioners in both the holistic and conventional camps, so choosing a practitioner is very important. Your impressions matter. Educate yourself by reading about the philosophy of the practitioner and about the treatment itself. If you have friends who have used practitioners you might be interested in, ask them about their experiences. Ask them to ask their friends and colleagues. You may choose a therapy because it has been recommended by a friend, or you may feel intuitively that a certain therapy will be 'right' for you.

If you are not familiar with non-conventional practitioners or don't have a reference you trust, you may want to go to a holistic health center where a variety of therapies are available. You might be able to have an advisory session with a staff member who would suggest therapies that might work well for you.

It is a good idea to shop around. Find out what works for you in terms of the personality and expertise of the practitioner, your comfort level with the treatment, and your level of trust in the practitioner him/herself. If you are uncomfortable with a practitioner, don't use him or her! Finding the right practitioner for you is subjective, and it's a good idea to listen to your instincts. Is their office clean or dirty? Do you feel comfortable in the office? Do you get the sense that they have good quality care and administrative processes to support the care given? Does the practitioner listen to you or does s/he have his/her mind somewhere else? Do you feel like they care about your concerns? Accept that you might not (and probably won't) find what works for you right away. Be patient, try different things that appeal to you or that you see as having some potential for healing. Questions you can ask in *Looking for the Right Practitioner* for you are listed in the appendix.

Do not expect to be cured by anyone else. Practitioners are guides to help you discover your *own* healing power and support you by giving helpful nudges along the way. You need to understand what is happening in your care and make choices about it on a general level, but the depth of your understanding about how the treatment works is up to you. That is another reason why trust in your practitioner is paramount. You will not know everything they know, and at some point you have to trust that they know what they are doing. You are always in charge in the sense that you have the choice of participating or not in your own healing. There is a balancing act when working with any practitioner between personal responsibility (understanding what is going on) and trust (being okay with not understanding everything that is going on).

When you are preparing to embark on the journey of finding a practitioner, be clear on what you do not want in a person or practice. Then develop some criteria about what you do want. Pick up flyers and holistic magazines in your local health food stores and bookstores, ask friends for their referrals, and keep your eyes open.

It is worth repeating that it's perfectly acceptable, and in fact crucial, that you discontinue treatment with anyone with whom you are not comfortable. It is also okay to change practitioners and you should try different practices. As one practitioner told me, a student takes more than one class and on your healing journey you will try more than one healing practice. The days of sticking to one practitioner (the family doctor) for most of your life are gone. Being straightforward about making different choices is great! You are expected to want to try different healers and different healing approaches.

Regardless of the setting in which you receive treatment (practitioner office, healing center, or hospital) do not be intimidated by anyone. The receptionist, nurse, practitioner, and other health care providers are all there to take care of you, whether they act that way or not. Follow up, think of questions beforehand and write them down so you will not forget them (i.e. explain my condition, what exactly does the treatment consist of, what can I expect, why should I do or take something). Sometimes health care providers might forget what they are there for (particularly when they are rushed or under stress), which is to help the person right in front of them, not the person ahead of or following them. Questions you can *ask during your visit* with any practitioner are listed in the appendix *Meeting with Your Practitioner*. It is not necessary to choose between conventional and alternative care. Although it may take some searching, we can choose conventional practitioners who believe in and understand holistic therapies and will be able to direct us to appropriate holistic practices. We can also choose holistic practitioners who will work with conventional practitioners. If either refuses to work with the other, find another practitioner. Your well-being is at stake.

Integrated care can be found in a variety of settings. There are individual practitioners who have some understanding of both conventional and alternative practices, there are healing centers with different kinds of practitioners, and there are hospitals and managed care organizations that provide (limited) access to both.

Health centers are groups of practitioners providing their services in the same place. Medical doctors usually direct or work alongside with holistic practitioners. In actuality practitioners rarely work as a team. It is up to you, the consumer, to make sure each practitioner knows, and hopefully understands, what other practitioners are doing. Most health centers seem to operate under a 'medical' model, where the physician is the authority.

Sometimes it becomes necessary to seek treatment in a hospital. That can be much scarier than treatments at a health center or outpatient facility where you get to go home when you're done. Hospitals can be frightening, dis-empowering experiences. The next section is about hospitals that are striving to be thoroughly healing institutions.

Holistic Hospitals

I created the term holistic hospitals to refer to institutions that provide integrated, patient-focused care. Holistic hospitals are focused on the well-being and comfort of the patient. Physicians are open to holistic, life-strengthening treatments in conjunction with allopathic, disease-fighting treatments. The emphasis is on healing the whole person rather than on fighting a particular disease or sickness. Care is given in a supportive rather than a toxic environment. Visitors are encouraged and supported.

In such a hospital modern medicine would be provided flawlessly (resulting from a functioning quality management system); health professionals and staff would be compassionate (because the hospital is a good place to work and cares for its employees); and patients would be completely supported in their own healing (due to innovative practices such as open visiting hours, the availability of kitchens and beds for family and close friends, nutritious foods, and the use of therapies such as massage, visualization, meditation, acupuncture and homeopathy).

While I do not yet know of any hospitals that have fully developed this concept, there are places working toward this. The resource listing provides descriptions of hospitals and health centers that I would want to know about if I were in need of such care.

The quality of medical care that a hospital provides is only one component of the healing experience. The range of healing approaches available and the extent patients (and their families) are involved in the healing process are also critical to the healing process. Patient-focused hospitals are developing programs to provide patients with better care and more autonomy. They are striving to create healing, nurturing environments and to involve patients and the patients' families in the healing process. Providers of patient-centered care have found the programs to be cost-effective. Data are available about a hospital's reputation, medical outcomes, death rates, number of board certified staff, and the ratio of registered nurses to beds. (See, for example: *Consumers' Guide to Hospitals*, 202/347-7283.) But how are *compassion* and *humanity* to be measured? Hospitals which claim to be patient-focused are good places to start your personal investigations.

Of course, the best hospital in an emergency is the *closest* hospital. However, even if you are already in a hospital you can still use this information to enhance your healing experience. Asking questions ahead of time will help you make the best choice when you have time enough for a *choice*. Hospital stays are anxiety-producing. Asking questions can relieve some of that anxiety, so even if you are worried about being a nuisance, speak up. You are allowed to make requests and ask questions, and there is reason to believe that patients who do speak up will have better healing experiences.

Hospitals are beginning to support non-conventional and holistic practices such as acupuncture, massage, nutrition, and music therapy. Even people who are skeptical about the effectiveness of holistic approaches believe that they are not harmful when practiced in conjunction with conventional medicine. At the very least they will add to the patient's comfort, and that in itself will aid the healing process.

Patient-centered or focused care is not necessarily holistic, but aims at making the patient's hospital stay as comfortable and empowering as possible. There might be classical music playing in the background, or available on CDs for patients. Soft, healing colors are reflected in the rooms, the hallways, and pictures on the walls. 'Pet' therapy may be available, using animals to comfort patients and accelerate the healing process. Full-spectrum lighting, believed to be health enhancing, is often used. The 'nurses station' is accessible and inviting. Patients wear their own clothing, sleep on soft sheets, and decide for themselves when they will get up in the morning.

There may be a private kitchen for the patients and their visitors to use to cook meals or make snacks. There may be video movies available to watch in a lounge or possibly in VCRs in the rooms. Medical charts are displayed and patients are partners in being responsible for their charting. There are no visiting hours because friends and family are welcome any time. Patients and family members receive extensive education about the disease(s) and how to support the healing process. Information is freely shared about diagnosis and on the proposed treatments and possible alternatives. The patient is in charge and the staff is there to inform, accommodate, and support the patient.

In patient centered hospitals, advanced medical technologies are available and integrated with the supportive comforts. Studies have shown that patients who are in pleasing environments, who feel in control, whose pain is adequately managed, and who are involved in their care have better medical results. Some of the studies supporting these findings are described in an article by Janice Hopkins Tanne in *American Health* (April 1993). Patient centered care is partially an attempt, based on these studies, to manage costs and provide more effective care.

Health Care Insurance

Many people have anxiety and confusion around the subject of health care insurance. Many very intelligent people feel completely illiterate when it comes to insurance and claim forms, and for good reason! Caring about insurance is necessary because medical care is so expensive. You want to have as much choice as possible, and if anything requiring acute or emergency care should ever happen, you want the best care available. You wouldn't ever want to be deprived of comfort or excellent attention because you didn't have the money to pay for it.

The basic options are:

1. **Insurance:** You pay for insurance and you pay for your health care. You are reimbursed a certain percentage (usually 80% once your deductible is met) of covered expenses.
2. **Preferred Provider Organizations (PPOs):** You pay for membership in the PPO and then pay a reduced cost for covered expenses and certain providers within their network of 'preferred providers'. You may also be reimbursed, at a lower percentage, for covered expenses provided outside of their network.
3. **Health Maintenance Organizations (HMOs):** You pay for membership in the HMO and almost all of your expenses within their network are covered.

HMOs are unlikely to cover providers outside their network. The advantage of insurance is greater choice; the advantage of HMOs is that you know how much you will be paying each month. PPOs are somewhere in the middle, offering more choice than an HMO but perhaps somewhat less than insurance. Compare your options (various insurance plans, HMOs or PPOs) based on coverage, expense, and convenience. Another way to get information about different health policies is to talk to insurance brokers. You can ask brokers for letters of reference from their clients.

Remember, plans with higher deductibles will have lower premium costs, other things being equal. Be clear on what is covered and how you get reimbursed for covered expenses. Look at the amount of co-insurance you are responsible for paying, and whether or not there is a limit on your out-of-pocket expenses. Ask for guidelines, in writing, about what kind of providers and treatments are covered and under what conditions. Ask them if they pay for alternative care, and if the practitioner has to be a medical doctor. You could also ask if you need a referral to see an alternative provider, how many visits are covered, and how much is reimbursable.

Many people have access to health coverage through their employers. If you do not work, are self-employed, or work for a business that does not provide health coverage, then you would need to purchase your own insurance. When purchasing insurance, one option is to take advantage of group rates available through plans offered by groups you already belong to or would consider joining. I wouldn't recommend buying insurance as an individual if you can help it. It is very expensive and your benefits are limited.

Almost everyone belongs to at least one group from which a group policy may be purchased. Look into groups such as your college alumni club, trade associations, social clubs, Chambers of Commerce, unions, or other groups with which you are affiliated. There are groups you can join and then take advantage of the group health insurance coverage.

Keep in mind that group plans vary in quality and the membership fee for joining the group may be high enough to outweigh potential health insurance savings. Your local library should have a book with information about associations and you might look there for other associations you either belong to or could join.

Although few insurance plans explicitly cover alternative care, it is still possible to get some alternative treatments covered. Many plans will cover any service provided by an MD or under an MD's supervision. It is sometimes possible to get or find a physician to prescribe holistic care. As in most endeavors, be persistent. Find practitioners you like and develop a rapport with them before you are sick. Educate them about alternatives and find out what they need to do to make a referral. Make their job as easy as possible.

The most important reason for health insurance is to cover catastrophic care, emergencies or acute illnesses that require expensive treatments or hospitalization. If this is the only reason you are buying health insurance, then it would be wise to choose a plan with a large deductible and pay for non-covered care yourself (referred to as out-of-pocket expenses).

Your deductible is the amount of money that you must spend before your covered expenses will be reimbursed. For example, if you have a $500 deductible, you must incur (and submit your claims for) $500 worth of expenses before they will start reimbursing you. The next dollar you spend on covered expenses, after spending $500, will be reimbursed, at whatever level is stipulated in your policy. Usually they will pay 80% of covered expenses.

Regardless of what kind of health coverage you have, you need to be persistent and vocal. Ask a lot of questions, keep good records and follow up. Make copies of everything you submit to your insurance company and submit claims even if you don't think they will be accepted. My attitude is, why not try and get reimbursed? The worst that can happen is they say it is not a covered benefit.

I keep two files for claims: pending and resolved. When I receive reimbursement from my insurance company, I take my copy of the claim out of the pending file, staple the check stub onto it, and file it in the resolved pile. Every month or so I call my insurance company (I am now on a first name basis with my contact there) and ask her what the status is with my claims. She may tell me she has not received it (in which case I mail her another copy), or she forgot about it (in which case I make a note of that and keep it in the pending file), or that she paid the provider instead of me (in which case I have to call the provider and get my money from them because I already paid them). Tracking the status of my claims has saved me hundreds of dollars.

Getting Started on Your Search

There are many excellent resources for finding alternative treatments for all kinds of disease states. There are research services (Planetree for example) and there are practitioners who will explore options for healing and discuss them with you. Associations and educational institutions will often provide referrals, at no charge.

The New Medicine that Dr. James Gordon writes about is a collaboration between practitioners and the person who is healing him/herself. It is about fueling the healing energy within us. We no longer have to choose between conventional and alternative practitioners. We can learn how to take responsibility for listening to our own guidance and fully participate in our own healing.

4

CHAPTER FOUR: DEFINITIONS OF TREATMENTS (CONTRIBUTED BY HEALTH CARE FUTURES) *

Approaches such as acupuncture, massage, breathwork, herbal medicine, and homeopathy are alternatives to what we in the U.S. call conventional, Western, mainstream, or allopathic medicine. Many of these alternative treatments are derived from ancient healing systems such as Ayurveda and Chinese Medicine systems which are many thousands of years old. For example, while Acupuncture may be nontraditional to us in the West, it is a traditional and conventional treatment in most Asian countries and has been evolving in that part of the world for over 5000 years. Allopathic medicine by contrast has been around a relatively short period of time.

The National Institutes of Health funded the Office of Alternative Medicine (OAM) in 1992. The Congressional mandate establishing OAM stated that the purpose is to 'facilitate the evaluation of alternative medical treatment modalities' for the purpose of determining their effectiveness and to help integrate treatments into mainstream medical practice. The OAM does not serve as a referral agency for alternative treatment modalities or individual practitioners.

Through the OAM's Exploratory Centers for Alternative Medicine Research, universities, clinics and practitioners receive small grants which cover research into a variety of treatments. Some of the current (1997) Exploratory Centers are the following:

1. Bastyr University, Seattle WA: AIDS Research Center.
2. University of Minnesota Medical School and Hennepin County Medical Center, Minneapolis, MN: The Center for Addiction and Alternative Medicine Research.

---

* Health Care Futures offers workshops, consultation, and lectures about complementary/alternative medicine. Contact information is found in the resource listing under the Educational Organizations/Programs heading.

3. University of Texas-Houston Health Science Center: The Center for Alternative Medicine Research in Cancer.

4. University of California, Davis: Center for Complementary and Alternative Medicine Research in Asthma, Allergy and Immunology.

5. University of Virginia: Center for the Study of Complementary and Alternative Therapies (CSCAT).

6. Stanford University: Complementary and Alternative Medicine Program at Stanford University (CAMPS).

7. Rosenthal Center for Complementary and Alternative Medicine (RHRC): The Center for Complementary and Alternative Medicine Research in Women's Health.

The Office of Alternative Medicine has listed 150 different therapies which fall into the category of Alternative Medicine. The major modalities, or practices, can be classified into 3 primary categories: Physical, Psychological, or Energy Therapies. Many, but not all, alternative therapies are discussed in detail in the following pages.

Physical Therapies work obviously and directly on the body in a very physical way both outside and internally. Examples are: Osteopathy, Chiropractic, Herbalism, Nutritional Therapy, Massage/Bodywork, Yoga and Aromatherapy.

Psychological Therapies help the body through the mind and the emotions. Examples of psychological therapies are: Counseling, Psychological therapy, Hypnotherapy, Relaxation therapy, Meditation, Guided Imagery/ Visualization and Biofeedback.

Energy Therapies are based on Eastern ideas of health and disease, and are based on the idea that illness is the result of an imbalance or an interruption in the body's natural energy or 'life force' at a very fine or subtle level. Examples are: Homeopathy, Acupuncture, Therapeutic Touch, Acupressure, Shiatsu, Reflexology, Reiki, Sound, Light, and Color Therapy, Kinesiology and Spiritual and Psychic Healing.

Two of the most well known ancient medical systems are Ayurveda and Chinese Medicine. Each of these complete systems encompass treatments from physical, psychological, and energy therapies.

Ayurvedic Medicine

Ayurveda is a system of preventive medicine and health care which teaches that all living things composed of elements and energies must be in perfect balance to be healthy. Ayurveda emphasizes equilibrium, a balance of mind, body and spirit. The focus is on the health of the body not on disease.

Ayurveda comes from two Sanskrit root words, Ayus or 'life', and Veda which means 'knowledge' or 'science'. Ayurveda is usually translated as 'the science of life.' A more literal translation would be 'the knowledge of the life span.'

Dating back to India over 5000 years ago, Ayurveda is the oldest medical system known, with its ancient texts covering every branch of medicine. Ayurveda has its roots in ancient Indian civilization and Hindu philosophy. It has been an important influence in the development of all other Oriental systems (i.e. Tibetan and Chinese Medicine). The original source of Ayurveda is the holy scriptures of the Vedas and the texts known as the Samhitas.

Theory

In Ayurveda, human beings are viewed as a microcosm of the universe. The human body and the universe are seen in terms of the 5 elements: space, earth, fire, water and air corresponding to the five senses of hearing, touch, taste, sight and smell. In Ayurveda the functioning of the body is controlled by spiritual forces linked to physical substances. Life force is 'prana' in Ayurveda, chi or qi in Chinese medicine. A person's individual constitution, prakruti, is determined by the dosha, or metabolic body type. All humans are composed of the three doshas, Vata, Pitta, and Kapha, but in most people, one dosha will predominate. The doshas are linked with specific energies and organ systems and are present in every life form. A preponderance of one type of energy over another is what determines our constitution and influences our personality. Vata, Pitta and Kapha are the predominant doshas. There are sub-doshas as well.

Vata dosha is composed of air and space. The seat of Vata is the colon. Vata is connected with the nervous system. The qualities of Vata dosha are COLD, leading to cold hands and feet, dislike of cold climates; MOVING, giving good or bad circulation; QUICK, ability to pick up new information quickly which is also quickly forgotten, poor long-term memory, good imagination, restless activity, mood swings, fast speech and scattered thoughts; DRY, dull skin, scant or moderate sweat, subject to eczema or psoriasis; and ROUGH, can have rough skin and course textured hair. The positive psychological traits of Vata dosha are imaginative, sensitive, spontaneous, resilient, and exhilarated.

Pitta dosha is composed of fire and water. The seat of Pitta is the small intestine. Pitta is responsible for metabolism and is equated with the body's heat and with digestion in general. The qualities of Pitta dosha are: HOT, leading to warm, flushed skin, hot sensations in the stomach, liver and intestines, fondness for cool food and drink; SHARP, leading to a sharp mind and often sharp speech, also excess acidity in the body and oversecretion of stomach acids; MOIST, leading to profuse perspiration, hot, sweaty palms, aversion to humid summer weather; SOUR-SMELLING, leading to bad breath, sour body odor and possibly bad-smelling urine and feces. The positive Pitta psychological traits are intellectual, confident, enterprising and joyous.

Kapha dosha is comprised of the elements of earth and water. The seat of Kapha is the chest. The themes of Kapha are structure and moistness. The qualities of Kapha are HEAVY, leading to obesity, heavy digestion, oppressive kind of depression; SWEET, leading to weight gain or diabetes if too much sweetness is added to the body; STEADY, leading to self-containment, steady nature, needing little outside stimulation; SOFT, leading to soft skin and hair, soft manners, a soft look in the eyes and an undemanding approach to situations. Psychological characteristics of Kapha are calm, sympathetic, courageous, forgiving and loving.

Symptoms

In Ayurveda, six stages of disease are identified. The first three are invisible and can be tied to either the mind or the body; the last three carry overt symptoms that can be detected by both the patient and doctor. Each stage represents a loss of balance, but the appearance of the loss of balance changes as the process continues. The six steps are:

1. Accumulation: the process begins with the build-up of one or more doshas.
2. Aggravation: the excess dosha accumulates to the point that it starts to spread outside the normal boundaries.
3. Dissemination: the dosha moves throughout the body.
4. Localization: the wandering dosha settles some where it does not belong.
5. Manifestation: physical symptoms arise at the point where the dosha has localized.
6. Disruption: a full-blown disease erupts.

Each of the three doshas has specific signs of imbalance: VATA exhibits worry, anxiety, short attention span, impatience, depression, insomnia, low appetite, constipation, intestinal gas, weight loss, arthritic joints, and loss of energy. PITTA has self-criticism, irritability, temper, criticism of others, skin rashes, ulcers, excessive thirst, bad breath, and rectal burning. And for KAPHA, signs are mental inertia, depression, slow movements, oversleeping, greed, sinus congestion, bloating, aching joints, limb heaviness, weight gain, diabetes, allergies, and asthma.

Consultation

An extensive history is taken from the client inquiring into likes, dislikes, sleep patterns, daily activities, food preferences, etc. Most helpful to the physician is the completion of a Mind/Body Questionnaire which asks the client specific questions related to each dosha, thus enabling the client and the physician to determine the course of treatment. This information is added to the physical data gathered (pulse and tongue diagnosis).

The Ayurvedic physician uses the pulse diagnosis and often the tongue inspection to determine the client's nature, predominant dosha, sub doshas and precisely where the imbalance is in the body which is causing the symptoms. With the pulse diagnosis the physician feels the quality of the three predominant pulses, and is thereby able to determine where to proceed in recommending treatment.

Treatment

Treatment in Ayurveda is totally individualized based on the person's body type and the location of the imbalance. In Ayurveda it is felt that disease occurs due to an accumulation of ama in the body. Ama is residual toxins in the body either from undigested food, undigested emotions, pollutants in the air, herbicides or preservatives in the food we eat or impurities in the water we drink.

Ayurveda offers the client a cleansing purification program called Panchakarma which literally translates as 'the five actions.' Panchakarma involves a complex series of steps tailored to the body type and the location of the imbalances to eliminate ama from the body and to ignite the digestive fire, agni. Panchakarma also serves to rejuvenate the cells once toxins are removed from the body. Panchakarma is recommended once a year for a week at a minimum and preferably three times a year (best at the turn of Fall, Winter and Spring).

Chinese Medicine

Chinese Medicine consists of acupuncture, moxibustion, herbal medicine, acupressure massage, cupping, therapeutic exercises and advice on diet and lifestyle. It is based on the principle of internal balance and harmony and teaches that when there is balance between all the internal organs, the body, the mind, and the external environment, there is good health. When the state of harmony and balance breaks down there is disease. Disharmony is the source of most disease.

Traditional Chinese Medicine has existed for at least 2000 years. The earliest Chinese Medicine text, 'Yellow Emperor's Canon of Internal Medicine', thought to have been written 500-300 B.C., is still used today.

Theory

In Oriental Medicine the body isn't viewed as a mechanical assemblage of parts nor are there rigid distinctions made between the body, mind and spirit. The client is viewed as a functionally integrated system and disease is seen as a condition affecting all aspects of the person, physical, mental and spiritual. Chinese Medicine uses the concept of universal energy or 'life force.'

Vital energy known as 'chi' or 'qi' is said to be the basis of all life. In the human body, the chi circulates through the body via 14 major energetic pathways called 'meridians'. Their existence can be detected electrically but can't be seen with the naked eye. Most of the meridians connect to one of the major internal organs and the chi is said to power the organ and enable it to function effectively.

Chinese Medicine believes that chi is regulated by interdependent forces of yin and yang which govern all living things. Yin qualities are typically coolness, weakness, hollowness and darkness, opposite the yang qualities which are heat, strength, solidity and light. A person's constitution or the nature of the disease may be described in terms of the yin/yang balance.

57

Chinese Medicine believes that the body is made up of 5 basic elements – wood, water, earth, fire and metal. It teaches that all 5 must exist in good balance in the body. If one of the elements is stronger than the others, the body will become unbalanced and the result will be disease in the body. The 5 elements are affected by the seasons, the weather, diet, and the emotional state. All these factors must be considered in diagnosis and treatment.

Physical Therapies

OSTEOPATHY AND CRANIAL/SACRAL OSTEOPATHY

Osteopathy is a manipulative treatment that works on the skeleton, connective tissue, and muscles of the body for the purpose of pain relief, improved mobility and health restoration. Osteopaths believe humans function as a complete working system with the body structure, organs, systems, mind and emotions all interrelated and mutually interdependent. Problems affecting one part of the structural body upset the balance of the entire body and the emotions. Chiropractic and Osteopathy are the most common forms of the manipulative therapies practiced today and are the only forms of this type of therapy which originated in the U.S. Osteopathy is a more complete system of medicine than is Chiropractic. Doctors of Osteopathy are able to perform the same functions as allopathic physicians, i.e. perform surgery, prescribe drugs and treatments.

Andrew Taylor Still founded osteopathy in 1874. He was initially trained as an engineer, later as an allopathic physician. He was displeased with the brutality and lack of scientific basis in medicine. He determined that stimulating the body's natural powers of self-healing would be the best approach. He became aware that many illnesses resulted from lack of alignment of the body's structures. Manipulation could restore the balance and cure illness. In 1930 William Garner Sutherland, a follower of Andrew Taylor Still, developed a specialized technique which is now called cranial/sacral osteopathy.

Theory

'Structure governs function' is the basic principle of modern osteopathy. An adjusted framework relieves strain on the body parts and helps the body systems to run smoothly so the body can heal itself.

The specialty of cranial/sacral osteopathy believes that the bones of the skull can be manipulated and retain some pattern for movement even in adulthood. Bones that move could be susceptible to dysfunction. Compression of the skull could have severe mental/physical effects. Dr. Sutherland discovered that the cerebrospinal fluid surrounding the brain and the spinal cord fluid had a rhythm which could be called the 'breath of life' because the rhythms appeared to be affected by the rate and depth of breathing. He found he could alter the rhythm of the flow by gently manipulating the skull. Any disturbance to the cranial bones can disturb normal motion of the bones and the cranial rhythm which ultimately affects the function in other body areas.

Symptoms Benefiting from Osteopathy

Osteopaths treat the same wide range of conditions which allopathic physicians treat. The following symptoms among many others experience relief from osteopathy: symptoms of direct trauma, headache, painful sinuses, decreased jaw mobility, tinnitus, residual effects of meningitis, some digestive and gynecological problems, back injuries, arthritis, body structure aches and pain.

In children, osteopaths have particular success dealing with ear infections, developmental delays due to cranial compression, hyperactivity, infant feeding problems, colic, poor coordination, sleep problems, learning difficulties and asthma.

Consultation

The osteopathic history is extensive, followed by an assessment of the body frame and posture. The doctor then takes every joint through the range of motion gradually increasing motion until the full range of movement is achieved. This is called active movement testing. Passive movement testing is accomplished by feeling the body's response to the movements of sitting, standing, walking, and so on. In a cranial/sacral osteopathic office, attention is paid to breathing, alignment of the cranial bones, to the hips and to the pelvis.

Treatment

Regardless of the field of Osteopathy the client chooses, the entire body is treated. A wide range of manipulative techniques are used depending on the part of the body requiring attention. Tight muscles are released so the body fluid may flow freely, and the blood and lymph systems work well. Touch may vary between low velocity, gentle, slow touch, to flexing and massage of joints and soft tissue. In cranial/sacral osteopathy, the practitioner begins by working the whole body to tune into the network of connective tissue. Next, various holding patterns of the head and neck are used with the practitioner applying light pressure. Fine, sensitive touch is applied to many areas of the body, but mostly the sacrum and the cranium. The idea is to resolve any compression or dislocation of the cranial bones, especially if any other part of the body is felt to be affected by compression or distortion.

CHIROPRACTIC

Chiropractic is technically described as the diagnosis, treatment and rehabilitation of conditions that affect the neuromuscular system. Chiropractic can diagnose and treat disorders of the nerves, muscles, bones and body joints, from headaches to ankle problems to the back.

Chiropractic derives from two Greek words meaning done by hand. Chiropractic is the most common form of manipulative therapy in the U.S. and is used for 94% of manipulative treatments. It is estimated that 15 million patients per year use chiropractic care.

Therapeutic manipulation of the body has ancient roots. Hippocrates (5th century B.C.), Aesklepiades (c.100

B.C.), and Galen (2nd century A.D.) all used some form of manipulation and it was common among physicians until the 18th century.

In 1895, Daniel David Palmer (1845-1913), a Canadian magnetic healer who was originally a grocer, felt a calling from his spiritual beliefs to find the 'cause for all diseases.' He discovered that 'displacement of any part of the skeletal frame may press against nerves, which are the channels of communication, intensifying or decreasing their carrying capacity, creating either too much or not enough functioning, an aberration known as disease.' He called his method of manipulation 'adjustment' and this method led to the establishment of a form of treatment known as chiropractic.

He began his practice in Canada by treating his office janitor for deafness by realigning the small bones in the spine. Word spread about his success and he eventually moved from Canada to Davenport, Iowa. The first Chiropractic school opened in 1895, the same year W.C. Roentgen invented the X-Ray machine which is used frequently today for making spinal assessments.

Theory

The nervous system is the master system of the body, and the spine is crucial to optimum health. When the back is functioning efficiently, the body is self curing. Chiropractic feels the spine is integral to 3 functional elements of the human body:

1. It surrounds and protects the spinal cord.
2. It supports many muscles.
3. It consists of an entire series of linked bones and has therefore many joints.

Any damage, disease or structural change of the spine (misalignment, called a subluxation) can affect the health of the rest of the body and manipulation can improve structural problems, like sciatica or effects of injury, and help with conditions like asthma (by easing the chest muscle tension). Palmer used spinal adjustment to treat disease, discovering that by gently moving misaligned bones back into place he could treat illness and avoid surgery and drugs.

Symptoms benefiting from Chiropractic

Chiropractic care is recommended for treating a variety of injuries, pain and illnesses. Some of these include: lower back pain, sciatica, neck and shoulder pain, tension headache, chronic leg, arm and hand pain, TMJ pain, pinched nerves, tingling and numbness in the extremities, PMS, ulcers, asthma, allergies, infertility, hypertension, anemia, respiratory problems, sports injuries, sprains and strains. Chiropractic should not treat osteoporosis, bone cancer, rheumatoid arthritis, broken vertebrae, conditions from severe circulatory problems, broken bones, acute infections and trauma.

Types of Chiropractic

1. **Network Chiropractic** uses light tapping and touching motions that increase relaxation and energy and often has reported psychotherapeutic effects, i.e. release of stored memories.

2. **Natural Upper Cervical Chiropractic Association (NUPPA)** is a school of thought that feels the brain stem is the most important part of the nervous system. It uses adjustments to correct misalignments of the atlas, the first cervical vertebrae. Misalignment of the atlas can cause back muscles to contract abnormally, misaligning the rest of the spine, causing lower back muscle pain. Relaxation of the musculo-skeletal problem will be beneficial for all organs and muscles.

Consultation

Diagnosis of the problem is performed through an extensive history review, observation of the client and a hands-on exam. X-Rays are used to gain an understanding of the underlying bone structure. Urine and blood samples are sometimes included. Also included is the study of the mobility and agility of the spine and of each of the patient's joints in the legs, neck, shoulders and arms to establish the range of motion of every vertebral and joint segment. This assessment is performed on the treatment table.

Treatment

Treatment is determined by the client's problem, age, body build, general health and pain levels. Where appropriate, the treatments consist of very precise adjustments to the spinal segments or the individual vertebrae to restore flexibility to stiff and painful joints, to reduce stress on neighboring joints and reduce reactive muscle tension and pain. Chiropractors concentrate on the localized problem and not on doing massage.

Chiropractors use special manipulative techniques:

1. Mobilization: moving a joint as far as it will comfortably go within the range of motion.
2. Manipulation: shifting of the joint further with one of a variety of techniques.

Hot and cold packs are frequently used to reduce pain and swelling depending on the injury as is a TENS (Transcutaneous Electro Neural Stimulation) unit. TENS works through the placement of electrodes to the tender area which blocks the message of pain to the brain, stimulates endorphins and causes relief of the sensation of pain.

Exercises are often recommended to improve posture, avoid future injury, stretch the back muscles and increase spinal mobility. Chiropractors do not prescribe drugs nor perform surgery. Today Medicare and Medicaid programs cover chiropractic care and 85% of insurance companies cover chiropractic services as well. Chiropractic treatment is often used in conjunction with acupuncture, massage, homeopathic remedies, aromatherapy, light and sound therapy and Chinese medicine.

NUTRITIONAL THERAPY

Although Hippocrates, the father of medicine, wrote extensively about dietary therapy, modern medicine (except in the case of diabetes and heart disease) has only recently begun to acknowledge the role nutrition plays in our lives. Good nutrition works on a therapeutic and preventive basis. What we eat is influenced by our culture, religion, lifestyle and personal preferences. Although it is often an illness which causes us to evaluate our diet, more and more Westerners are becoming involved in nutritional awareness for the preventive benefits.

Dietary Considerations

Andrew Weil, MD, the widely recognized advocate for Integrative Medicine, and author of *Spontaneous Healing* and *8 Weeks to Optimum Health* offers numerous suggestions for planning a healthy, preventive nutritional future. A sampling of the suggestions are:

1. Reduce animal protein as much as possible. Add fish high in omega-3 fatty acids such as salmon, sardines, kippers and mackerel to the diet.
2. Eat plenty of fruits and vegetables, including cooked, dark, leafy greens such as beet and mustard greens, chard, kale and collards.
3. Increase the intake of dietary fiber by replacing refined grains with whole grains whenever possible, brown rice instead of white rice and whole grain breads instead of white bread.
4. Reduce the intake of white sugars and sweets.
5. Decrease the intake of highly processed, packaged foods.
6. Decrease caffeine intake in the form of coffee and cola and replace it with herb teas or green tea. Green tea has cancer-preventive and anti-bacterial effects, as well as cholesterol lowering effects.
7. Increase cardio-vascular system protectors: garlic, onions, hot peppers, green tea, shiitake mushrooms, salmon and sardines, and ginger.

8. Avoid artificial sweeteners containing saccharin, aspartame and products made with them.
9. Read labels of foods and discard oils containing partially hydrogenated oils and foods containing them.
10. Discard oils which are smelly, old or rancid. Eliminate margarine, cottonseed oil, solid vegetable shortening and products made with them.
11. Use extra-virgin olive oil for cooking, salads, etc. Olive oil contains mostly monounsaturated fat, far better than saturated or polyunsaturated fat.
12. Eliminate products containing artificial coloring and chemical additives.
13. Make an effort to keep the total fat intake to 20-25% of calories, and saturated fat intake as low as possible.
14. Increase the intake of cruciferous (cabbage family) vegetables, such as broccoli and cauliflower due to their significant anti-cancer properties.
15. Be aware of the water which you are drinking. Consider a water filtration system to guard against heavy metals, organic chemicals, bacteria, nitrates, herbicides, parasites, etc.
16. Consider purchasing organic fruits and vegetables, grown free of herbicides, pesticides and fungicides.

Fasting serves the purpose of ridding the body of toxins said to accumulate from the wrong diet so that the body can begin to function at its optimum. Two days duration is an appropriate time for self-regulated fasts. Water is taken in unlimited quantities during the fast. Return to eating gradually, slowly re-introducing foods in the following order: raw fruits, salads, whole grain foods, protein sources, and then dairy products. Fatty, sugary, refined carbohydrates, coffee, tea, colas, alcohol and tobacco should be eliminated totally. Frequently during a fast, in addition to water, juices are added. It is recommended that the fruit and vegetable juices be organic and freshly squeezed.

Body Intelligent Tips

In his book, *Perfect Health,* Deepak Chopra talks about Body Intelligence Tips (BITS). These are helpful hints to be considered in any nutritional program which can add significantly to the enjoyment of every meal and help expand the satisfaction the body derives from the eating experience. How you eat is as important as what you eat. Including the use of sight, smell, hearing and touch in addition to taste is the only way to completely make use of the mind/body connection.

The BITS are:

1. Eat in a settled atmosphere.
2. Never eat when you are upset.
3. Always sit down to eat.
4. Eat only when you are hungry.
5. Avoid ice-cold food and drink.
6. Don't talk while chewing your food.
7. Eat at a moderate pace, neither too fast nor too slow.
8. Wait until one meal is digested before eating the next (intervals of 2-4 hours for light meals, 4-6 for full meals).
9. Sip warm water with your meal.
10. Eat freshly cooked meals whenever possible.
11. Minimize raw foods - cooked food is much easier to digest.
12. Do not cook with honey.
13. Drink milk separately from meals, either alone or with other sweet foods.
14. Experience all 6 tastes at every meal (sweet, sour salty, bitter, astringent and pungent).
15. Leave one-third to one-quarter of your stomach empty.
16. Sit quietly for a few minutes after your meal.

MASSAGE/BODYWORK

Massage and bodywork are effective and wide-ranging therapeutic tools, incorporating touching, stroking, kneading and pressure which work on both a physical and psychological level. They can enhance general well-being, health, and vitality and offer an excellent way to relax the mind, body and spirit and bring relief from the everyday stressors of the modern world.

In the 5th century B.C., Hippocrates wrote 'the way to health is a scented bath and an oiled massage every day'. Massage is one of the oldest forms of bodywork and was a part of many ancient cultures including China, India, Greece, Arabia and Persia. It was first practiced in China over 5000 years ago.

Most modern methods of massage come from Swedish massage developed by Per Henrik Ling, a Swede who visited China during the 19th century. He created his own form of massage drawing from what he experienced in China. Currently there are about 80 different types of massage and bodywork and only about twenty of them are more than 20 years old.

There are 3 major categories of massage and bodywork:
European/Swedish/Chinese/Japanese: Swedish is the most popular type of European massage, using long gliding strokes, kneading, stroking and friction. This is the type of massage used most frequently in the U.S. in spas and health clubs. Amma is the earliest massage practiced in China now practiced around the world. Amma means 'massage' in Chinese. In the first half of the 20th century Amma massage was performed by blind people in China. Amma uses a wide variety of massage movements over the entire body including kneading, stroking, vibration, and circular pressure techniques. The massage treatment uses fingers, elbows, hands, and knees for treatment. Amma uses the energy points to balance and unblock yin and yang energy that may be impairing health. In Amma massage the client remains fully clothed and no lotions or oils are used.

Deep Tissue: Structural integration (rolfing), Aston Patterning, and Hellerwork.

Movement Integration: These methods teach better ways to move the body efficiently and comfortably using highly structured movement sequences with particular emphasis on the head positions to decrease stress. Examples of movement integration are: Feldenkrais, the Alexander Technique, and Trager, the latter which combines light tension releasing movements with a series of gentle, painless, passive movements that increase the freedom of movement.

Symptoms benefiting from Massage and Bodywork

The benefits of massage are numerous. Conditions which respond best to massage are circulatory and heart disorders, hypertension, headaches, hyperactivity, insomnia, back and neck pain, anxiety and depression, stress and its related disorders, and the release of knotted muscles and spasms. The client senses an increased sense of well-being, relaxation, calm, peace and tranquillity with massage.

YOGA

Yoga is an ancient philosophy of health and well-being which has had an important influence on mind body medicine in the Western world. Yoga derives from the Sanskrit language. It means 'union' or 'joining' and implies the harmony of mind, body and spirit. Yoga is one of the ancient religious schools of the Hindus and has evolved over several centuries. Ancient archeological evidence suggests it may be 5000 years old. It is considered a sister science of Ayurveda and deals with the science of the spirit, and Ayurveda with the science of the body. The modern masters of yoga (yogis) are Iyenga, Sivananda and Jois.

Theory

In the West, we think of Yoga as only a series of postures, but in reality it is part of an entire philosophical system which seeks enlightenment, oneness with the Supreme Being.

The best known forms of Yoga are:

HATHA: In the West it is the form known to be associated with physical movements or postures (asanas). Hatha comes from 2 Sanskrit words, 'ha' which refers to the sun, and 'tha' which refers to the moon. Proper breathing is essential to correctly execute the asanas and deal with the mental core needed for the meditation practice.

In Hatha yoga it is believed that breath (prana), or 'the life force', is blocked when we are ill, during emotional or physical stress or when toxins are in our food, water or in the air we breath. Prana, 'the life force', is drawn in with every breath and carried throughout our bodies. Controlling the breath is called 'pranayama' which means 'regulating the life force.'

There are approximately 80 postures (asanas), each of which is part of a group that benefits various body systems, although all benefit the entire body and mind. Asanas alternate between activity and rest. Each asana is composed of the movement to reach the pose and a phase of holding the pose. The postures stimulate and help regulate the nervous, circulatory and endocrine systems.

RAJA: This yoga primarily involves meditation. It focuses on the mental aspects of yoga rather than the physical postures.

ASHTANG: This yoga combines aspects of both Hatha and Raja yoga. The basis of the practice is linking the Hatha postures into flowing movement which use the mind to affect the breath control, periodically divided by a number of physical 'locks.'

KUNDALINI: This yoga is referred to as the 'coiled serpent' at the base of the spine. Movement of Kundalini Energy can activate the chakras and cause changes in consciousness.

TANTRIC: Tantric yoga includes the postures and breathing technique of Hatha yoga. It also seeks to use Kundalini energy and the body's subtle energy centers to achieve heightened awareness. Tantric yoga is often associated with awakening sexual pleasures.

Symptoms Benefiting from Yoga

Yoga is often used as a therapeutic tool and recommended for injury and illness recovery. The most pronounced effects of yoga are improvement with: anxiety and depression, chronic illness, asthma, rheumatism, arthritis, stress and stress-related disorders, insomnia, fatigue, circulatory and hypertensive problems, neck and back pain, headaches and respiratory disorders. Yoga is also used as a complementary therapy for cancer patients and is a useful therapy for strengthening abdominal muscles, shoulders, legs, back and the neck.

AROMATHERAPY

Aromatherapy is the beneficial use of essential oils derived from a wide variety of plants, distilled from the roots, bark, leaves, resin, flowers, and rinds. Aromatherapy derives from the French word 'aromatherapie' coined in the early 1900s by French chemist Rene-Maurice Gattefosse, who considered the use of the essential oils of plants another branch of herbal medicine. Jean Valnet, a French MD, used essential oils to treat wounded soldiers in World War II and began investigation into their healing properties. His work helped establish aromatherapy as a valid treatment approach in France. Although aromatherapy is still considered a nonconventional treatment in the U.S., it has gained wider acceptance in Great Britain and elsewhere in Europe among orthodox practitioners.

Aromatherapy is often used in conjunction with massage therapy, chiropractic, herbal treatments, nutrition, homeopathy and naturopathy. It can be used alone or as part of a treatment or preventive program.

Theory

As the science of olfaction and the art of aromatherapy

come together, the mystery around how aromatherapy works is disappearing. The nose, more than any other sense, has a vast vocabulary amounting to about 10,000 different odors. Odors which can be detected by the nose are first dissolved in the nasal tissue's moisture and then directly passed on to the hypothalamus in the brain by specialized olfactory calls. These olfactory cells are the only ones in the entire body directly exposed to the air. The hypothalamus is the 'brain's brain', responsible for regulating the functions of sleeping, waking, sexual arousal, temperature, thirst, hunger, blood sugar levels, growth, and the emotions of anger and happiness. To smell anything is to send an immediate message to the brain's regulating center and from there to the rest of the body.

Electrochemical messages are then sent to the limbic system, the brain's emotional processing area, and the release of neurochemicals is triggered. Messages are also sent to an area called the hippocampus, the part of the brain responsible for memory. This physiological connection is the reason why odors and smells trigger such vivid memories so rapidly. Perfumes, and garden and kitchen smells all trigger a sense of deja vu.

Neurochemicals have a wide variety of effects, such as either promoting relaxation or stimulation. Messages are then sent to other body areas which result in a change in mood or energy shift or a sense of draining tension.

When essential oils are on the skin, the molecules are absorbed through the hair follicles and pores. They get into the bloodstream through the capillaries and circulate through the body. Oils act on organ systems, and on all cells and body fluids. Mucous membranes are also affected by essential oils, which makes conditions of the lungs and nasal passages receptive to treatment with these substances, either through inhalation or by application on the skin in the form of a compress or massage oil.

Symptoms Benefiting from Aromatherapy

Aromatherapy is used effectively to reduce stress and anxiety, alleviate insomnia, treat acne, cellulite and aging skin, muscular and rheumatic pains, digestive disorders, PMS, menopause problems, postnatal illnesses, and skin conditions. Aromatherapy is also used for the relief of common infections like colds and the flu. Some essential oils are physically therapeutic while others possess antibacterial, antiseptic or anti-inflammatory properties.

Essential oils must be extracted from the plant. The process is different with every plant depending on where the oil in the plant is most concentrated. Some oils are distilled with the process of heating and cooling, other oils are squeezed or scraped out of the plant part. It takes varying amounts of a plant to make the different oils, e.g. it takes 2300 pounds of rose petals to make 1 pound of rose oil. An extraction process of this magnitude explains the considerable expense of many of the essential oils.

Essential oils are generally diluted in cold-pressed vegetable oils such as almond, soybean, grapeseed, avocado or wheat germ oil. These are called 'carrier oils'. Essential oils may contain hundreds of naturally occurring chemicals and are classified by their volatility, the speed by which they evaporate when exposed to the air. Volatility is linked to the effects on the body. Oils with increased volatility have energizing, stimulating effects, used to promote a state of mental alertness and concentration. Essential oils with decreased volatility are used to promote calm, peaceful states.

Essential oils are highly concentrated and can cause irritation if applied directly to the skin, and should therefore in most cases be diluted in carrier oils. Also aromatherapy should be avoided altogether in a pregnancy with complications. During a normal pregnancy, aromatherapy should be avoided during the first trimester and after that should be instituted only under the supervision of a certified aromatherapist.

Essential oils are selected for the effect desired. They are to be used singly or with no more than three oils together. There are many ways to experience the benefits of aromatherapy. Essential oils can be placed: in bath water, under running hot water, on a handkerchief under the nose, on the pillow, in a vaporizer with the head held over a bowl under a towel, in an inhaler, in an electrical diffuser (called an Aromastream), on a heated piece of ceramic (called an Aromastone), in massage oil, on a cottonball on the radiator, on a light bulb ring, in an atomizer used for household plants to spray the room with a favorite fragrance, and some can be used directly on the skin.

Ten Useful Oils (derived from Norm Shealey's work)

Oil	Effect
Chamomile	Calming – also useful in treating pre menstrual tension/pain, indigestion, hay fever, acne, eczema, and other sensitive skin conditions.
Eucalyptus	Antiseptic – also useful with premenstrual pain, indigestion, hay fever, acne, eczema, and other sensitive skin conditions.
Geranium	Mildly Astringent – also used for treating cuts, sores, fungal infections, eczema, bruises, depression, fluid retention, low energy, as an insect repellent, and for treating mild skin problems.
Lavender	Mildly Astringent – also used to treat headaches, other aches and pains, wounds, bruises, insect bites, oily skin, acne, swelling, mild depression, and for calming insomnia.
Rose	Antiseptic – also used for treating a sore throat and sinus congestion, swollen eyes, puffiness, blood circulation problems, insomnia, depression, reduced libido, and premenstrual pain/tension.
Rosemary	Mild Stimulant – also used to treat physical and mental fatigue,

	forgetfulness/absentmindedness, respiratory problems, and to soothe rheumatic aches and pains.
Sandalwood	Antiseptic – also used on dry, cracked, chapped skin, acne, as calming relaxation during meditation, and as an aphrodisiac.
Marjoram	Mildly Analgesic – also used to treat menstrual pain, headache, sore throat, insomnia, thrush, and acne.
Jasmine	Antidepressant – also treats depression, strengthens contractions during labor, and is an aphrodisiac.
Neroli	Mildly Sedative – also treats insomnia, anxiety, nervous depression, acne, backache, and premenstrual tension/pain.

Psychological Therapies

MEDITATION

Meditation is one of the most frequently suggested stress-reduction tools. It is a way of contacting the inner energy that powers the natural processes of healing and self-realization. Meditation offers an increase in equilibrium between the rational left side of the brain and the creative right side, causing an increase in the brain's range of operation. Meditation has many different forms, some of which are not dependent on a particular spiritual system while others are associated with and taught by followers of Eastern religions.

Mantra Meditation: uses a word or phrase, repeated in the mind, to help the learner quiet his/her thoughts and reach a deeper level of consciousness. Mantras are selected on the basis of the learner's temperament and occupation. Some mantras are selected on the basis of the person's birth date using Vedic Astrology. Transcendental Meditation and

Primordial Sound Meditation are examples of Mantra meditations.

Mindfulness Meditation: the person pays nonjudgmental moment to moment attention to the changing objects of perception and cognition.

Breath Awareness: observation of or following the breath as the person repeats the cycles of inhalation and exhalation (i.e. Zen Meditation).

Prayer: the use of a rosary, prayer beads, or just repetition of simple prayers.

Other: walking meditation, performing other pleasant activities, concentration on the heavens, etc.

All forms of meditation have certain characteristics in common. They all work to quiet the mind, help us become aware of our breathing, help us focus on the present moment, not the past or the future, and provide us with a time-out from the world.

Symptoms Benefiting from Meditation

The benefits of meditation are numerous. In Jon Kabat Zinn's Stress-Reduction Clinic at the University of Massachusetts Medical Center, a study found that after eight weeks of meditation training, 60% of the patients had a 50% reduction in their pain. At the same Center, in a study of 225 patients with chronic pain who were taught mindfulness meditation, 60% reported moderate or greater improvement in pain reduction after a four year period.

Other benefits reported are a slowing of the heart rate, lower blood pressure, decreased muscle tension, decreased stress hormone production, increased alpha brain wave production, increased awareness, decreased panic disorders, decreased chronic pain, decreased feelings of anxiety, anger and depression and increased happiness, self-confidence, effectiveness, and general well-being.

How to Meditate:
* Find a quiet location without distractions.
* Sit quietly in a chair or on the floor.
* Close your eyes for 5-10 minutes (to start).
* Pay attention to your breathing by following each breath, each inhalation and exhalation through your nose, or focus on an object in your mind such as a flower, scene in nature, a religious symbol, or concentrate on a favorite poem or verse, or if using a mantra meditation, repeat the mantra to focus awareness away from your thoughts and active mind.
* Repeat this process twice daily, gradually working up to 15-20 minutes meditation in each session.

GUIDED IMAGERY/VISUALIZATION

Guided Imagery/Visualization produces a response in the body and uses the power of the mind. Imagery is a natural means of communication between your body, mind and spirit. Specific images, sounds, and smells are also used in addition to words. Guided Imagery/Visualization techniques are often used with relaxation, biofeedback, hypnosis, and medical and behavioral treatments.

Guided Imagery and Visualization are emerging as important mind/body medicine techniques. Imagery is used in the business world and in education to increase self-confidence and reduce stress. Sports psychologists advise skiers, basketball players and others to picture successful performance in their minds before they execute plays. In one survey of elite athletes, 99% reported using imagery techniques to enhance their performance.

Theory

Imagery uses the imagination to focus and work with an issue directly. It is a way of talking to the body. It establishes a dialogue between the client and the illness. Imagery is a very important way of bringing information from the unconscious to the conscious mind. Dialogue images may reveal hidden motivations and fears.

Guided Imagery can be used as a complementary treatment for almost any illness, injury or condition, both chronic and acute. Guided Imagery may alleviate symptoms or side effects of disease.

Benefits from the use of Guided Imagery and Visualization
* increase in self-awareness, self acceptance and self worth
* when combined with scientific technology and modern medicine, imagery can facilitate a patient's comfort and healing
* decreases the severity of side effects of treatments and medication
* increases the effectiveness of treatments
* increases the sense of control over treatments (especially for cancer treatments)
* decreases the fear some treatments may produce (i.e. chemotherapy and radiation)
* offers increased control for acute and chronic pain, both physical and psychological
* decreases anxiety and fear
* can be an important tool in understanding a disease process in the body and may lead to powerful insights into what the disease means to that person
* gives focus and direction to a client's imagination by using specific words and suggestions
* increases a sense of control over an illness
* alleviates the inflammation and pain associated with arthritis and other chronic conditions
* often used in hypnosis and is shown to increase blood sugar, stomach secretions, inhibit GI (gastro intestinal) activity and alter skin temperature

Treatment
Guided Imagery sessions usually last between ten and thirty minutes in acute care settings and more than 60 minutes in other contexts. Practice is key to developing deep levels of

insight. Imagery allows the practitioners to help the client make perceptual and behavioral changes which promote healing. Guided Imagery/Visualization is not a substitute for conventional treatment, but used as an adjunct.

Guided Imagery is carried out by helping the client to reach a relaxed state which leads to the mind and body becoming quiet, receptive and inwardly focused, allowing images to flow more and more freely. A practitioner uses progressive muscle relaxation, encouraging the client to first tense up, then relax every muscle group, starting with the feet and moving up. Another method used to induce a state of relaxation is a simple countdown, counting down from 10 to zero. At zero the client is completely relaxed and refreshed. Once relaxed, that state can be deepened through breathing exercises. The practitioner might say for example, 'Pay attention as you inhale and exhale, notice if your breathing is shallow or deep. Notice any changes in its quality or in the number of breaths per minute.'

This is not recommended for psychotic patients already experiencing too many images who are unable to differentiate between those they choose to envision and those that plague them involuntarily. The dialogue technique can bring up powerful insights which can be frightening, confusing and even depressing.

Energy Therapies

HOMEOPATHY

Homeopathic practice is based on the three principles of Dr. Hahnemann: the Law of Similars, the principle of the minimum dose, and prescribing for the individual. Treating the patient as a whole person is probably the most important part of homeopathy. Homeopathy feels each person is an individual and must be treated as such.

The name homeopathy comes from the Greek word homoios meaning 'like' or 'similar', and pathos which means suffering. It simply means treating like with like. The principle is an ancient one dating back at least to the time of Hippocrates, who wrote in 400 B.C. 'Through the like, disease is produced and through the application of the like, it is cured.'

The beginnings of homeopathy are credited almost entirely to one person, Samuel Christian Hahnemann (1755-1843). He was a physician and chemist born in Meissen, Germany who was greatly distressed by the medical practice of his day. Instead of following the usual practices his fellow physicians prescribed for their patients, such as bleeding, blistering, cupping and purging, he prescribed exercise, a nourishing diet and pure air.

Hahnemann was fed up with the lack of a rational basis for therapeutics. He started experimenting with pharmaceuticals due to an interest in the effects of drugs on the body. Why were they given? What did they do to the system? How did they act? He lived at a time when experimental and scientific pharmacology did not exist. Pharmacology was in such disrepute that the situation was of concern to every MD. Hahnemann complained that if he sent a prescription to 10 different pharmacies, he would receive back ten different preparations, each having a different effect on the system. In 1810, Hahnemann published his most important work, the Organon of Homeopathic Medicine.

In 1820, homeopathic medicine was introduced to the U.S. by an immigrant from Denmark, Hans Gram. For many years homeopathy was a respected health care system that coexisted with a variety of schools of thought. The formation of the American Institute of Homeopathy, the first national medical society in the U.S. in 1844 directly caused the founding of the AMA in 1846. Most new homeopaths in the U.S. were orthodox MDs who abandoned their practices due to dissatisfaction with medicine as it was being practiced in the U.S. at that time.

The AMA was openly hostile throughout the 19th century. Although once considered part of mainstream medicine, homeopathy eventually became suppressed by medical practitioners in the U.S. During the period 1850-1880, conventional MDs were sanctioned from dealing with homeopaths, actions were taken to restrict homeopath's practices, and the AMA demanded homeopathy be removed from state medical societies.

By 1930, homeopaths were almost extinct. U.S. interest in homeopathy has risen dramatically since the 1970's with the American public's interest in alternative medicine. Homeopathy is today used widely in India and throughout Europe.

Theory

Hahnemann believed that a drug which produces symptoms of a disease in a healthy person will cure a person who has that disease. He proved this after using himself as his subject to study malaria. He did not have the illness, but when taking quinine (a substance from the cinchona bark) he began to manifest symptoms of malaria. From this experiment he developed his theory of the Law of Similars, referred to as 'like cures like.'

Hahnemann's experiments led him to view the body as a whole, not a collection of separate parts. He believed that the 'vital force', the body's innate intelligence, was working to maintain the body's harmony when a person is healthy, or in a state of balance. He felt that symptoms which occur during an illness are the body's way of working to restore balance. Symptoms are viewed as part of the creative process not to be suppressed.

Hahnemann's experiments also led to his Law of Potentization (also called The Law of Infinitesimals). From his experiments he came to the realization that as he diluted the medicinal substances he was testing, effectiveness was enhanced. Thus the higher the dilution number (as noted by the 3x, 6x, 30x etc. on the bottle) the more times the substance has been diluted. The higher dilutions prove to be stronger and, in most cases, the most effective. These minute substances are called homeopathic remedies. Low potencies like 3x or 6x are used for chronic conditions and higher potencies like 30x or 200x are used for acute conditions and illnesses such as colds, flu or trauma. Hahnemann believed that it was the energy or 'vibrational pattern' of the remedy, rather than its chemical content that stimulates the healing by encouraging the body's own healing force.

Symptoms Benefiting from Homeopathy

Homeopathic remedies are good for everyone: the general population, babies, pregnant women and the elderly. Homeopathy can treat almost any complaint, acute or chronic, physical or psychological, although its effectiveness seems to depend on the individual.

Examples of conditions helped by homeopathy are: indigestion, childhood illnesses, gallstones, depression, burns, sports injuries, allergies, stress, travel sickness, peptic disorders, kidney disorders, hyperactivity, cold sores, bursitis, irritable bowel syndrome, indigestion, asthma, skin problems, arthritis, heart disease, and nicotine, drug and alcohol withdrawal.

Consultation

A homeopath studies a person's temperament, personality, emotional and physical responses, activities engaged in, food likes and dislikes, family history, past illnesses, lifestyle, diet, sleep patterns, ability to face responsibility, whether the person has cold feet or hands, and so on.

Treatment

Homeopathic remedies come in the form of granules, liquid, powder, tablets, or small pills which are taken one-half hour before or after eating or drinking. The client should experience a change in his/her condition within a few days. Treatment may require only one or two visits, but chronic conditions take longer to treat and heal. The remedies are to be taken only for as long as needed. Remedies can be taken with conventional medicine.

There are over 3000 homeopathic remedies, which are usually referred to by their abbreviated name, e.g. Mercurius solubilis becomes Merc. sol. and Arsenicum album becomes Ars. alb. These homeopathic remedies are harmless dilutions of minerals, plant extracts and other natural substances.

ACUPUNCTURE

Acupuncture is one of the major components making up the practice of Chinese Medicine. It represents an Eastern way of looking at the world and nature and expresses a philosophy that has evolved over centuries into a many-layered system of examination and diagnosis. Acupuncture works by stimulating points on the body surface that affect the physiological functioning of the whole body or a specific system. Jesuit missionaries from France gave acupuncture its name. It derives from the Latin, 'acus' for needle and 'punctura' for puncture.

The history of acupuncture dates back a long way. An ancient Chinese story is told about wounded warriors who sometimes recovered from chronic diseases after being shot with arrows in combat. In the 6th century B.C. medical texts describe acupuncture. And in 400-200 B.C., The Yellow Emperor's Canon of Internal Medicine was compiled. This was the first book on acupuncture.

Over thousands of years acupuncture has grown to become the standard medical practice of the Chinese people. It is also the primary care method for hundreds of millions of people throughout Asia.

Acupuncture and Chinese Medicine tradition spread throughout Asia in the 6th century. In the 17th century, Jesuit missionaries from France came into contact with and carried its first beginnings to Europe. It disappeared from Europe as a practice, only to reappear in 1938. When MaoTse-tung's revolution happened in 1949, he sent 'barefoot doctors' into the countryside of China armed with simple tools for acupuncture. Currently both traditional and Western Medicine are practiced in China.

In 1971, New York Times correspondent in China, James Reston, had an appendicitis operation in China. The Chinese doctors used only acupuncture and a local anesthetic during the surgery and he was conscious for the entire procedure. His post-operative pain was also managed only with acupuncture. Acupuncture's move into Western Medicine began with the news of this experience.

Theory

The theory behind acupuncture is that there is a vital energy in the body called Qi (chi) flowing through the meridiens or the energy channels in the body. Signs and symptoms manifest when disharmonies develop that block the flow of energy through those meridiens.

Qi circulates through bodily channels or meridians called Jingho. These form a circuit of the body, through which the internal organs are connected to one another. There are 12 main channels traversing the body's trunk, as well as arms, legs and head. In classical theory, there are 350 acupuncture points on the meridians of the body. However, over time the number of known points has increased to over 2000.

Discovery of brain endorphins in the 1970s stimulated the interest of Western Medicine in acupuncture. Researchers conducted a number of experiments that explored the role of endorphins in acupuncture anesthesia. Acupuncture increases the production of endorphins. Acupuncture also increases the levels of other essential body chemicals, including serotonin and cortisol. It has also been postulated that acupuncture may tap into the body's electromagnetic properties.

Symptoms which benefit from Acupuncture

Acupuncture is very effective for pain treatment. This effectiveness is very well documented in over 100 studies confirming acupuncture use for pain relief. In one literature review, researchers found up to 80% of people with back pain, headache and other assorted painful conditions were helped. Other researchers found that individuals who had suffered migraine and tension headaches for 20 years or more reported greater relief from acupuncture than from conventional therapy.

Acupuncture is also very effective for treating a myriad of conditions such as: joint problems, specific organ involvement, mental and emotional illnesses, childhood illnesses, eye problems, myopia in children, cataracts, acute conjunctivitis, digestive disorders such as hyperacidity, acute and chronic duodenal ulcers, hiccups, constipation and diarrhea, bones and muscle disorders, frozen shoulder, sciatica, osteoarthritis, general lower back pain, insomnia, arthritis, depression, headaches, and anxiety.

Evidence also exists to show that acupuncture can help overcome addictions to alcohol and drugs. For cancer, acupuncture is used as a complementary therapy along with herbal and nutrient treatment. It has the positive side effects of aiding patients in dealing with the unpleasant reactions (nausea and vomiting) to chemotherapy and radiation.

Consultation

Acupuncture diagnosis is made by the practitioner questioning the patient about presenting complaints and about other seemingly unrelated areas such as sleep, digestion, elimination, emotions, sex drive, menstruation patterns and energy level. The patient's tongue is examined for size, shape, color and coating. Condition of the client's eyes, fingernails, skin, hair and face overall are also carefully examined. The practitioner also palpates the pulse for 28 different qualities while the patient assumes 6 different positions. This information is compiled and a pattern of disharmony is arrived at which leads to the diagnosis.

Treatment

Needle insertion with very thin, sharp, sterile needles is quick and virtually painless. One treatment may be considered enough, although four to seven treatments is average. Acupuncture may be performed on hands, feet, legs, forearms, abdomen, back and forehead. Once inserted, needles may be twirled or wiggled to be inserted deeper. Patients are asked to relax with the needles in place for 20-30 minutes. Most people report a sense of relaxation and an increased sense of well-being following an acupuncture treatment. Although rare, infections have been reported from reused needles. These infections include exposure to HIV and hepatitis.

Types of Acupuncture
Traditional: Preventive treatment, used for maintaining optimum health, practiced with other modalities like herbalism.
Acupuncture for anesthesia: Gaining wide acceptance in the U.S. and around the world. Localized pain can be treated and major operations have been performed with acupuncture for anesthesia.
Treating symptoms: Pain relief, concentrated on symptoms.

THERAPEUTIC TOUCH

Therapeutic Touch is a method of 'laying on of hands' for the purpose of transferring healing energy to the client. In Therapeutic Touch, the practitioner does not actually touch the client. Therapeutic Touch was developed in 1972 by Dolores Krieger, R.N., Ph.D. after seeing the work of Hungarian healer, Oscar Estabany, and studying with healer Dona Kuntz and other psychic healers. In the 1970's Dr. Krieger introduced a graduate nursing course on Therapeutic Touch at New York University. In 1979, Dr. Krieger wrote *Therapeutic Touch: How to Use Your Hands to Help and Heal.*

Therapeutic Touch has been taught to thousands of nurses and health care practitioners in the U.S. and in 38 countries. It is a part of the curriculum at 80 universities in the U.S. and abroad.

Theory

Therapeutic Touch is based on the belief that in a healthy person there is an equilibrium between inward and

85

outward energy flow. Illness is an imbalance in this energy field or disruption in the energy flow. The field of human energy, called bioenergy, extends beyond the skin, beyond the physical body. The goal of Therapeutic Touch is to restore balance to the person's energy field, thus allowing the person to recover his own healing powers.

Treatment

When doing Therapeutic Touch, healing is facilitated by using the practitioner's hands to consciously direct an energy exchange. The entire process lasts approximately 25 minutes.

With the client sitting in a chair or lying on a bed, the practitioner first synchronizes his/her energy to that of the client. During the treatment the practitioner holds his/her hands apart, one on each side of the client. Concentrating on the client, the practitioner moves his/her hands slowly toward the client's feet, scanning the energy field for subtle bilateral differences. Differences in the feel of the energy field are cues to the practitioner of energy congestion. They are frequently found at sites other than an area of pain. The back is scanned first, the front last. The client remains fully clothed, because the energy field penetrates clothing.

Hands of the practitioner usually move or hover just one or two inches above the client's body and may be held on the body if the 'field' feels deficient or cold. By placing the hands over the body and moving in sweeping motions, the Therapeutic Touch practitioner unruffles the bioenergetic field of the body.

A skilled practitioner knows that a healthy balanced energy field has a symmetrical, smooth flowing texture. Signs of imbalance (congestion or deficiency) which a practitioner might experience include bilateral difference in temperature, texture, rhythm or energy flow. The practitioner seeks to balance the client's energy field so it feels uniform and flowing. This is done by warming a cool area, directing energy toward an area which seems diffused or empty.

Benefits of Therapeutic Touch

Therapeutic Touch induces a state of profound physical and often mental relaxation in patients. A spreading feeling of warmth or sometimes pleasant vibration is reported. In acute care settings following Therapeutic Touch treatments patients require less pain medications, describe greater pain reduction with and without analgesics, experience more rapid wound healing, experience longer periods of pain relief post-operatively which allow the patient to be more alert so he/she can be more actively involved in his/her own care. Clients also report decreased anxiety and a bolstered immune system function. The Office of Alternative Medicine is funding a study on Therapeutic Touch's effects on the immune system and response to stress.

ACUPRESSURE, SHIATSU, JIN SHIN JYUTSU

Acupressure has been practiced for centuries in Japan and China and uses the same energy points along the meridians as acupuncture with the purpose of promoting the smooth flow of energy throughout the body. In acupressure massage the acupuncture points are pressed and held for specific periods of time to correct any imbalance of the Qi (chi) energy that could cause illness or discomfort. These points are called Tsubos and are located along the meridians.

Shiatsu ('finger pressure') is a form of acupressure from Japanese tradition that uses points along the same meridians as straight acupuncture but involves rhythmic finger pressing or deep, gentle finger pressing that lasts for 3-6 seconds on every point. **Jin Shin Jyutsu,** developed by Jiro Murai, an early Japanese philosopher, is a gentle type of acupressure that involves long holding of the acupressure points for 1-5 minutes while meditating on the part of the patient to maximize the benefit to the body.

REIKI

The name 'Reiki' is itself a fusion of 2 Japanese words, Rei which means universal and Ki which means life force.

Reiki is pronounced 'ray-kee'. It is a form of healing based on tapping into the unseen flow of energy permeating all living beings. Practitioners believe that this life force is in all of us and that this energy is a healing power that properly instructed practitioners can tap into.

Reiki is an ancient Tibbetan Buddhist practice which transferred knowledge of its power from master to disciple. It was rediscovered by a late 19th century Japanese Christian minister named Dr. Mikao Usui in Kyoto, Japan. Usui sought through his studies, especially of Buddhism, to investigate the healing power of history's great spiritual leaders. Before his death, Dr. Usui initiated 16 others into the secret of Reiki, teaching them the master attunement.

Reiki was first brought to the U.S. in the 1940's by Hawayo Takata, a Japanese-American woman who studied under an associate of Dr. Usui in Tokyo. Reiki was made popular in the U.S. by Timothy A. McNamara of the Usui Center for Natural Healing in Denver. In the early 1980s, the Reiki movement divided and subdivided. There are now a half a dozen different versions of Reiki.

Treatment

Treatment by a Reiki practitioner is intended to promote physical, emotional and spiritual well-being. Clients remain fully clothed while the practitioner's hands are placed on specific body parts, starting with the head, transferring 'universal life energy' to the client.

Some Reiki practitioners don't touch the physical body but transmit healing to the surrounding area. Reiki can be used to heal the self or someone else. Reiki energy can be projected into the future or directed to a distant place. Results of treatment can be dramatic or general, steady improvement in health and well-being. Daily self-treatment is regarded as preventive, supporting emotional and spiritual growth.

Sound, Light, and Color Therapy

SOUND THERAPY

The ancient Hindus said 'the fundamental reality is sound.' Scientists tell us the world, from stars to atoms, quarks to planets, vibrates. Sound is vibration and everything in creation vibrates. Sound is one of our oldest healing tools. It has also played an important role in the religious and cultural rituals of every society. Tibetan monks have used 'overtone chanting' for thousands of years to treat illness.

The idea that music may be a key to healing the body and mind has occupied Western culture for thousands of years. The field of musical therapy, healing with music, voice and sound, is among the oldest and most holistic of medical approaches. Novalis, the 18th century German mystical poet, stated 'Every sickness is a musical problem. The healing, therefore is a musical resolution. The shorter the resolution, the greater the musical talent of the doctor'.

Pythagorus, the 6th century B.C. Greek philosopher, who today is credited as the founder of Western music therapy, sang calming melodies to his followers. These melodies were based on the principle that melody and rhythm, which originate in cosmic laws, restore harmony to our souls. He felt that music supports health and can produce 'the most beneficial correction of human manner and lives.'

Theory

The theory is that since everything in the universe is in a constant state of vibration, including the human body, even the smallest change in the frequency can affect the internal organs. The human ear can distinguish 1378 different tones within the vibrating range of 16-25,000 hertz (cycles per second). Many sounds exist outside the audible sound spectrum. Yale University scientists have determined that 6 visible planets, including the Earth, emit distinct sounds created by their magnetospheric waves (e.g. the sun comprises 80 different overtones).

Healing Effects

The healing effects of music and sound fall into three major categories:

1. Music can greatly improve the quality of life for people with serious illness, disabilities or depression, as well as those having surgical or medical procedures. Music is very effective for patients with Alzheimer's and Parkinson's disease and can facilitate restoration of movement, mental clarity or partial physical coordination. Music also serves as palliative therapy for autism, dyslexia, and chronic physical disabilities.

2. Music provides clarification and access to possible resolution of deep-seated psychological and emotional issues and underlying physical and mental conditions.

3. Music can facilitate soul-level spiritual insights and healing. An example of this is the use of music to ease the process of dying for the patient and the family members.

Today's therapists of sound ascribe to the theory that there is a natural resonance or note 'that is right for every part of the body and for every person. By directing specific sound waves to specific body areas, they can affect the frequency at which that part is vibrating and thereby restore it to balance and therefore health.' (Richard Leviton, Yoga Journal, Jan.-Feb. 1994)

Symptoms Benefiting from Sound Therapy

Sound is used to decrease pain and inflammation such as soft tissue damage, arthritis, fractures, sports injuries, rheumatism and back pain. Pain relief is due to the release of tension thereby producing balance in the body. Sound therapy is also effective in the reduction of anxiety and pain, as well as the increase in relaxation in the general population and also with very specific audiences such as women in labor. Music in the Recovery Room after surgery has been shown to help patients recover from their anesthetic more rapidly. Music has also been proven to assist developmentally delayed children and adults with speech development and sensory motor coordination.

Toning is the use of sound to create vibrations in the body. 'Om', the sound used in many meditation practices is an example of this. Continuing repetition of one long sound, usually a vowel is felt to be one of the fastest and easiest ways to reduce stress and stop 'mind chatter' that decreases focus and mental concentration.

Guided Imagery and Music (GIM)

Founded by music therapist, Helen Bonny, Ph.D., Guided Imagery and Music is a music-centered psychotherapeutic process. She describes GIM as a 'technique that involves listening to music in a relaxed state to illicit imagery, symbols and/or feeling for the purpose of creativity, therapeutic intervention, self-understanding and religious (spiritual) experience'.

LIGHT THERAPY

Like sound therapy, light therapy is one of our oldest healing tools. Our ancient relatives knew about the internal clock which influences how, when, and for how long we sleep, as well as energy and mood fluctuations throughout the day. This internal clock is called our circadian rhythm.

Theory

Light plays an important role in the way the hypothalamus functions. As light enters the eye, it is converted to electrical impulses which move along the optic nerve to the brain, thus triggering the hypothalamus. The hypothalamus works by means of neurotransmitters or chemical messengers. The hypothalamus, part of the endocrine system, helps coordinate the work of various body systems, i.e. digestive, circulatory, sexual function and the circadian system.

A photobiologist and light therapy researcher, John Nash Ott, believes poor lighting is bad for health and can adversely effect the body's ability to absorb nutrients. He believes that beneficial light must contain full wavelength, the spectrum occurring in natural sunlight. He concluded that many conditions such as cancer, mental and dental disorders are made worse by inadequate exposure to full spectrum light.

Exposure to full spectrum light has been shown to have positive effects with insomnia, PMS, migraines, hypertension, childhood hyperactivity, and decreased bilirubin levels in newborns. Studies have been performed which suggest that full spectrum lighting can play a role in the prevention of some forms of cancer, colds and sore throats in factory workers, improvement in school attendance and academic performance in students as well as a decrease in hyperactivity and behavioral problems.

Seasonal Affective Disorder (SAD)

Seasonal Affective Disorder, 'the winter blues', affects about 1% of the population (more women than men). S.A.D. is a seasonal related depression which seems to be connected to the production of melatonin by the pineal gland. The production of melatonin increases in the dark and decreases in the light. Melatonin is an essential hormone which plays a role in immunity and has a sedative effect which helps induce sleep.

Insufficient light passes into the light-sensitive pineal gland, the part of the brain controlling appetite, sleep, mood and sexual desire. The level of indoor light produces only about 1/10 of the illumination of a full day of natural light.

Symptoms of S.A.D. Benefiting from Light Treatment

Symptoms of S.A.D. include feelings of withdrawal and helplessness during dark periods of the year, depression, lethargy, carbohydrate craving, decreased sex drive, fatigue, and increased need for sleep.

Treatment

Treatment with full spectrum light, either sunlight or white light exposure for one to four hours a day proves to be effective in 85% of the S.A.D. cases reported. This can be accomplished with either going outdoors to sit in the sunlight, sitting near windows in light-colored rooms or having full spectrum light boxes installed into the home and office.

COLOR THERAPY

Normal daylight (sunlight) is filtered through the eye to produce the visible colors of the spectrum: red, yellow, orange, green, blue, indigo and violet. Ultraviolet and infrared light affect us even though we cannot see them.

Color is an energy form and each color stimulates different psychological and physiological changes. It is believed that as light is received and absorbed through the skin, it works on the nervous system to change the body's chemical balance. By adjusting specific colors we look at, physical mood and well-being are affected.

Scientific studies have confirmed that every cell of our body is made up of contracted light and because light responds to color, color therapy is directed at restoring cells to an even level of balance, stimulating any necessary healing process and improving overall spiritual and mental health.

On the subtle energy level, therapists work to influence the chakras, the 7 energy centers. Each chakra corresponds to one of the 7 colors of the light spectrum, starting at the base chakra with the color red, all the way to the violet at the crown chakra (top of the head). Green is said to influence the heart chakra and yellow the solar plexus.

Examples of the Effects of Color

RED   arouses the body, increases heart rate and brain wave activity, speeds up circulation.

PINK   has a calming effect, promoting relaxation and soothing the mind.

YELLOW   stimulates the memory and increases energy.

GREEN   mental uplift and relaxation. Green is often used in hospitals and nursing homes for its relaxing qualities.

BLUE   calming effect on adults and children, decreases blood pressure.

Leaders in the Integrated Medicine Field

Over the past five years, several physicians have become very visible in the arena of healthy lifestyles, natural healing and the mind body link, pointing out to us that there are other ways to look at our lives, our health and the choices we make regarding each of these areas. Physicians who have been at the forefront of Mind Body Medicine are: Deepak Chopra, Larry Dossey, Christiane Northrup, Dean Ornish, Bernie Siegel, Carl Simonton, and Andrew Weil.

Awareness of the mind body link got its first big boost in the U.S. with the 1979 publishing of *Anatomy of an Illness* by Norman Cousins, then editor of the Saturday Review. He contracted ankylosing spondylitis, a disease of the connective tissue. His specialists told him that they had never witnessed anyone recovering from this illness. His illness caused him to take a deeply searching look at his life, his stresses, and his priorities and then make major, far-reaching adjustments. He embarked on a course of action which entailed several points:

1. He had total involvement in decisions for treatment with his doctor. His opinion, his courage, and his tenacity as a patient were respected and encouraged.
2. Substitution of pain-killers with genuine belly-laughter from movies and television offered hours of pain-free sleep.
3. Focus on the positive emotions of hope, faith, love, and laughter.
4. Total belief that he would get well and the realization that thoughts and emotions in his mind were directly connected to mobilizing his body's own natural healing resources.

Norman Cousins went on to become an Associate Professor of Medicine at the University of California at Los Angeles and lecturer to medical students about his experience and encouraged research on the mind/body connection.

DEEPAK CHOPRA, MD

Deepak Chopra exposed the American public to Ayurvedic Medicine, the 5000 year old healing system incorporating mind, body and spirit from India. Although trained in Western medicine as an endocrinologist, Dr. Chopra has become synonymous with and probably the main standard bearer for Mind Body Medicine, as exemplified by Ayurvedic Medicine, which has gained an enormous following in this country.

Through Dr. Chopra's many books, tapes, international lectures, workshops and widely acclaimed PBS series, he has offered the public a unique view of health and illness, particularly the reasons we get sick and how our thinking contributes to the creation of the state of illness or wellness. Although initially aligned solely with Ayurvedic Medicine, Dr. Chopra uses an eclectic approach in his thinking, drawing on the wisdom of a variety of medical systems and encourages patients to recognize that Ayurveda is just one system of many which can help a patient.

In Ayurvedic philosophy, our body's natural and spontaneous intelligence is designed to keep us physically, emotionally and spiritually well. Meditation is an integral part of Ayurvedic treatment, and it is also part of prevention, and maintaining optimal health. Meditation is a vehicle by which we can come to a deeper understanding of our nature and eventually less identified with illness and disease. Dr. Chopra's most popular book titles are: *Perfect Health* (a great resource to Ayurveda); *Unconditional Life; Quantum Healing; Ageless Body, Timeless Mind; Seven Spiritual Laws of Success; Return of the Rishi;* and *The Return of Merlin.*

LARRY DOSSEY, MD

Larry Dossey, a physician from Texas, is a world authority on the beneficial effects of prayer on patient outcomes. He feels that prayer is one of the best kept secrets in medical science and that an enormous body of evidence exists that prayer works. This information, if recognized and honored, could change the way medicine is practiced and could also revolutionize our ideas about healing.

Dr. Dossey examines the evidence of prayer's effectiveness and explores the role of the unconscious in prayer, how prayers manifest through dreams and the dangers of believing that we can totally and consciously create our own reality. His writings reflect the changes he has undergone, starting from a place of believing that prayer was little more than superstition. After years of medical practice, he was stunned to discover scientific evidence of the healing power of prayer. His scientific worldview shaken, he embarked on 10 years of research on the relationship between prayer and healing.

Dr. Dossey lectures internationally. He is the former Chief of Staff of Humana Medical City Dallas and current co-chairman of the newly established Panel on Mind/Body Interventions, Office of Alternative Medicine, National Institutes of Health. He is the Executive Editor of the professional publication, Alternative Therapies in Health and Medicine. He has written the following books: *Space, Time and Medicine; Beyond Illness; Recovering the Soul; Meaning and Medicine; Healing Words;* and *Prayer is Good Medicine.*

CHRISTIANE NORTHRUP, MD

Dr. Northrup is a graduate of Dartmouth Medical School, and did her internship and residency in Obstetrics and Gynecology at Tufts New England Medical Center, in Boston. Since 1983 she has been assistant clinical professor of obstetrics and gynecology at the University of Vermont College of Medicine. She was the President of the American Holistic Medical Foundation between 1986 and 1989. She has been on thescientific advisory board of Natural Health Magazine since 1981. She co-founded Women to Women, an innovative Yarmouth, Maine health care center in 1986 that has become a model for women's clinics nationwide. She was co-president of the American Holistic Medical Society with Bernie Siegel, MD between 1988 and 1990. Dr. Northrup wrote *Women's Bodies, Women's Wisdom* in 1994.

Dr. Northrup is changing the medical mindset by educating women everywhere about their options, their alternatives, and their medical rights. She lectures and teaches internationally on all issues of women's health and wellness. In her practice she is achieving dramatic results with many of the frustrating female problems such as PMS, endometriosis, chronic vaginitis, fibroids, depression, breast cancer and eating disorders. She deals with the emotional issues underlying presenting symptoms and works with her patients to clear them. She deals head on with toxic emotions, toxic relationships, toxic beliefs and toxic attitudes, all of which impact women's emotional and physical health.

DEAN ORNISH, MD

Heart disease can be reversed by incorporating a vegetarian diet, exercise, stress management techniques, and group support meetings. After several years of data collection at eight U.S. Medical Centers using the Dean Ornish Program for Reversing Heart Disease, it has been proven that the Ornish Program can halt the progression of – and often reverse – coronary artery blockages without drugs, surgery or other medical interventions.

Dean Ornish, now at the Preventive Medicine Research Institute in Sausalito, California, began researching what was available in the literature about non-invasive treatment for coronary artery disease while still in medical school. Isolated studies about the effects of a low-fat diet, smoking cessation, and exercise existed but no researcher had pulled all these factors together into one study. Dr. Ornish did so and went on to have the first non-invasive program for reversing heart disease paid for by a commercial insurance. Mutual of Omaha became the first company to endorse the program, paying for a 24 or 30 day stay at the Ornish Center. Over the long haul, the Ornish treatment program is far less expensive than drugs and surgery, with lasting results.

The Ornish program requires that patients take responsibility for their health and exhibit a willingness to continue on a self-care program. The stress-management component includes yoga stretches, progressive relaxation techniques, breathing exercises, meditation and guided imagery. The group support meetings are called 'Opening Your Heart'. Dr. Ornish links a person's emotional well-being with his/her ability to reverse heart disease. Dr. Ornish has stated that he sees heart disease as a metaphor for the feelings of loneliness and isolation, the real heartaches so many people in our society feel in their lives. He believes that healing the body cannot be separated from the mind or the spirit. A vegetarian, low-fat diet is recommended for participants. Walking is the recommended exercise and the program advocates a one hour walk several times a week.

Given the success that the program has had in documenting that heart disease can be halted and reversed using the components of the program, Dr. Ornish is now preparing to take on other types of chronic illnesses to determine if those illnesses can also be halted or reversed. Dr. Ornish's books are: Stress, Diet and Your Heart; and *Dr. Dean Ornish's Program for Reversing Heart Disease*.

BERNIE SIEGEL, MD

Bernie Siegel, MD, a graduate of Colgate University and Cornell University Medical College, is a retired general pediatric surgeon. Dr. Siegel prefers to be called Bernie and describes himself as a cheerleader for life. His brand of medicine works at healing people not eliminating disease. Through the years, in his numerous books and workshops, he has focused on the emotional element needing healing in the patient with cancer or chronic disease. He employs Art

Therapy in his workshops, and his books show many examples of the drawings of patients who are giving life to their wishes, hopes, dreams, desires, fantasies, sadness and unresolved emotional conflicts which might be a key to healing their illness.

Dr. Siegel founded EcaP (Exceptional Cancer Patients) and through it offers practical tools to explore the role of hope, love, spirituality and unconscious beliefs in the healing process. He uses meditation, Art Therapy, laughter and play. He is now involved with humanizing medical care and medical education, making doctors and patients aware of the mind body connection. He also has an interest in combining spirituality through meditation and medical treatment. His books include the titles: *The Psychology of Illness and the Art of Healing; Love, Medicine and Miracles; Peace, Love and Healing;* and *How to Live Between Office Visits.*

O. CARL SIMONTON, MD

O. Carl Simonton, MD is an internationally acclaimed physician, medical director of the Simonton Cancer Center in Pacific Palisades, California, and director of the Psychoneuroimmunology intervention counseling program for Cancer Treatment Centers of America. Dr. Simonton is widely recognized for his pioneering research and treatment of cancer patients, focusing on improving the quality of life for individuals with advanced cancer using counseling techniques. He was prominent in his role in pointing out that cancer and other illnesses are often a symptom of unresolved emotional conflicts occurring on a deeper level. In addition to counseling, which forms the basis of the cancer therapy, and in addition to whatever conventional therapy the patient may be on, Dr. Simonton utilizes many other forms of therapy, such as Art and Music Therapy. Dr. Simonton is an international lecturer and author of *Stress, Psychological Factors and Cancer; Getting Well Again;* and *The Healing Journey.*

ANDREW WEIL, MD

Andrew Weil received an A.B. degree in biology (botany) from Harvard and an MD degree from Harvard Medical School. After completing an internship in San Francisco, he worked with the National Institute of Mental Health. Later, from 1971-75, as a fellow of the Institute of Current World Affairs, Dr. Weil traveled throughout North and South America and Africa, collecting information on drug use in other countries, medicinal plants and alternative methods of treating disease. From 1971-84, he was on the research staff of the Harvard Botanical Museum and conducted investigations of medicinal and psychoactive plants.

Dr. Weil is director of the Program in Integrative Medicine at the University of Arizona College of Medicine, Tucson, where he teaches alternative medicine, mind/body interactions and medical botany. He holds appointments as clinical assistant professor of medicine and clinical assistant of family and community medicine. Dr. Weil is also the founder for the Center for Integrative Medicine, a not-for-profit scientific and educational foundation dedicated to creating new paradigms of medicine for the 21st century.

A frequent lecturer and guest on talk shows, Dr. Weil is an internationally recognized expert on alternative medicine, medicinal plants, addiction, altered states of consciousness, and the redesign of medical education. Dr. Weil is the author of 7 books: *The Natural Mind; The Marriage of the Sun and Moon; From Chocolate to Morphine; Health and Healing; Natural Health, Natural Medicine; Spontaneous Healing;* and *8 Weeks to Optimum Health.*

5

CHAPTER FIVE: WHAT'S POSSIBLE?

"The current method of medical care will be outmoded within the next ten years. Hospitals will care for the seriously ill, and the majority of care will take place in decentralized community-based healing centers, staffed by licensed spa technicians (for massage and aromatherapy) as well as allopaths, nutritionists, acupuncturists, mind-body specialists, and movement therapists," according to Pamela M. Peeke, MD, stress physiologist, and assistant professor at the University of Maryland School of Medicine (Carol Isaak Barden, *Condé Nast Traveler*, May 1997).

Andrew Weil, MD, director of the Program in Integrative Medicine at the University of Arizona College of Medicine and best selling author believes that "a lot of hospitals will go bankrupt. My hope is that they will be resurrected as healing centers..., where people go for a week or so and learn how to eat, exercise, and use their minds to access their own healing power. This kind of treatment would be paid for by insurance". (Body Mind Spirit - Special Issue, 1997)

Holistic Community Centers

My interest in holistic health began in my early teens. I dreamt of starting a holistic community center which would address physical well-being, serve nutritious and tasty meals, be a magnet for fun social activities like dancing get-togethers, and provide information and resources supporting individual activism and empowerment. In college I researched holistic centers and tried to find out what it would take to start such a center. That was in the early 1980s – very few such centers existed. The only one I knew of was the Berkeley Holistic Health Center, in California. I spent a summer doing an internship with them, learning about how a holistic health center operates.

These holistic community centers would be places where people could receive a variety of services supporting their well-being. They would have practitioner offices, a healthy eating place, a resource library with an empowerment corner containing information about how to take action on a wide range of issues, a room for child care, and rooms for dancing, social events, and meetings. These centers are today becoming realities.

6

CHAPTER SIX: RESOURCE LISTING

This chapter contains listings for resources you can use to get answers to your questions.

In the first section are listings for getting **information** about various healing approaches:

Associations
Research Organizations/Services
Educational Organizations/Programs
Health Insurance
Publications
Web Sites

In the second section are listings for finding **places** to go for healing:

Clinics/Centers
Hospitals
Retreats/Spas

Section I: Information and Referral Sources

You can use these resources to get referrals and information about credentials for various practitioners.

Associations

Academy for Guided Imagery
Interactive Guided Imagery(SM)
Roy Johnston
E:mail: agi1996@aol.com
PO Box 2070, Mill Valley, CA 94942
(415) 389-9324 Fax (415) 389-9342
We provide a certification training program in Interactive Guided Imagery(SM) for Health Professionals.

Academy of Pain Management
3600 Sisk Road, Suite 2D, Modesto, CA
(209) 545-0754

Alliance/Foundation for Alternative Medicine
PO Box 59, Liberty Lake, WA
(509) 255-9246

Alternative Health Professional Society
2001 North Collins, Suite 101, Richardson, TX
(214) 644-5900

American Academy of Environmental Medicine
4510 West 89th Street, Suite 110,
Prairie Village, KS 66207
(913) 642-6062

American Academy of Medical Acupuncture
C. James Dowden
E-mail: KCKD71@prodigy.com
5820 Wilshire Boulevard, Suite 500,
Los Angeles, CA 90036
(213) 937-5514, (800) 521-2262; Fax (213) 937-0959
When you include SASE, they will refer you to AAMA members in your area.

American Academy of Osteopathy
1127 Mount Vernon Road, PO Box 750, Newark, OH
(614) 366-7911

American Apitherapy Society (Bee Venom Therapy)
Box 54, Hartland Four Corners, VT 05049
(804) 436-2708

American Art Therapy Association
1202 Allanson Road, Mundelein, IL 60060
(847) 949-6064

American Association of Ayurvedic Medicine
PO Box 541, Lancaster, MA
(508) 368-1818

American Association of Naturopathic Physicians
2800 East Madison Street, Suite 200, Seattle, WA
(206) 323-7610

American Association of Oriental Medicine
433 Front Street, Catasaqua, PA 18032
(610) 266-1433
They offer a list of acupuncturists who meet its
standards.

American Association of Orthopedic Medicine
5147 Lewiston Road, Lewiston, NY
(716) 284-5777

American Chiropractic Association
E-mail: amerchiro@aol.com
1701 Clarendon Boulevard, Arlington, VA 22205
(800) 986-4636; (703) 276-8800; Fax (703) 243-2593
Offers free referrals from 21,500 members who do
spinal adjustment and medically-oriented
supplemental therapies. All are licensed doctors of
chiropractic with over 5 years of post-graduate
training and internship through accredited
chiropractic colleges. The American Chiropractic

Association is a national non-profit professional health care association representing the majority of doctors of chiropractic in the U.S. The ACA mission is to enhance the philosophy, sciences and art of chiropractic, and the professional welfare of individuals in the field. The ACA services and programs include providing information pertaining to the chiropractic profession, educational requirements, research related to chiropractic efficacy, and the benefits of chiropractic inclusion in health insurance reimbursement plans, from both cost and wellness standpoints.

American College of Nurse-Midwives
1522 K Street Northwest, Washington, DC
(202) 289-0171

American Environmental Health Foundation
8345 Walnut Hill Lane, Suite 200,Dallas, TX
(214) 361-9515

American Foundation for Alternative Health Care
25 Landfield Avenue, Monticello, NY 12701
(914) 794-8181

American Foundation of Traditional Chinese Medicine
1280 Columbus Avenue, Suite 302, San Francisco, CA
(415) 776-0502

American Holistic Health Association
Suzan Walter, President
E-mail: ahha@healthy.net
(Web Page http://www.healthy.net/ahha)
(714) 779-6152
PO Box 17400, Anaheim, CA 92817-7400
A national clearing house for self-help resources promoting health and well-being. AHHA offers free resource and networking lists and an award-winning newsletter with self-help tools; AHHA is an all-

volunteer non-profit educational association. AHHA encourages personal responsibility, considering the whole person and whole situation, wellness lifestyle choices, and active participation in one's personal health decisions and healing process.

American Holistic Medical Association (AHMA)
6728 Old McLeam Village Drive, McLeam, VA 22101
(703) 556-9728
Membership includes all state-licensed holistically-oriented practitioners, such as physicians, chiropractors, naturopaths, nurses, psychologists, and dentists. They publish a referral directory ($5) for the U.S.

American Holistic Medical Association/Foundation
2002 Eastlake Avenue East, Seattle, WA
(206) 322-6842

American Holistic Nurses' Association
4101 Lake Boone Trail, Suite 201, Raleigh, NC
(919) 787-5181

American Institute of Ayurvedic Sciences
2115 112th Avenue Northeast, Bellevue, WA 98004
(206) 453-8022

American Massage Therapy Association
1130 West North Shore Avenue, Chicago, IL
(312) 761-2682; (800) 696-2682
They can help you find a local massage therapist.

American Naprapathic Association
5913 West Montrose Avenue, Chicago, IL
(312) 685-6020

American Oriental Bodywork Therapy Association
Glenndale Executive Campus, #510,
1000 Whitehouse Road, Boorhees, NJ 08043
(609) 782-1616

American Osteopathic Association
142 East Ontario Street, Chicago, IL
(800) 621-1773

Aromatherapy Institute of Research
PO Box 2354, Fair Oaks, CA 95628
(916) 965-7546

Associated Bodywork & Massage Professionals
www.expectmore@abmp.com
28677 Buffalo Park Road, Evergreen, CO 80439
(800) 458-2267; Fax (303) 674-0859
ABMP offers a free referral service for locating a
professional massage therapist or esthetician in your
area. Membership in ABMP provides the massage
therapist, bodyworker, and esthetician with excellent
professional liability insurance, training and product
directories, Massage & Bodywork magazine, and
many other benefits.

Association for Applied Psychophysiology & Biofeedback
10200 West 44th Avenue, Suite 304,
Wheat Ridge, CO 80033
Offers free referrals to over 1,500 practitioners who are
trained and certified in various modalities of
biofeedback therapy. Written requests only with
enclosed stamped, self-addressed #10 envelope.

Association for Network Chiropractic
Donald M. Epstein, DC, President
E-mail: ancoffice@aol.com
444 North Main Street, Longmont, CO 80501
(303) 678-8101; Fax (303) 678-8089
The Association for Network Chiropractic is an
international professional association composed of
healing professionals and lay persons sharing a
common vision for world healing. Key concepts are
that our participation in the world is in direct
relationship to our participation with our bodies, that

as each of us heal it assists the species and the global community, that a spine and nervous system free from mechanical tension assists in the expression of health and well being, that the Network approaches to chiropractic are important tools to assist individuals in achieving health and well being, that the body mind and body's natural organizing wisdom are in a partnership which needs to be respected and honored, and that our individual healing promotes global healing. The ANC publishes newsletters, conducts seminars, develops 'think tanks' and research projects supporting the advancement of this world vision.

Association of Health Practitioners
PO Box 5007, Durango, CO
(303) 259-1091

Association of Holistic Healing Centers
Margaret Irby, Ph.D.
E-mail: ahhcIrby@aol.com
PO Box 2367, Carefree, AZ 85377
(602) 488-5502; Fax (602) 588-1371
A non-profit membership organization supporting the creative development of health centers which offer integrated services (traditional and alternative) through teams of health care professionals for diagnosis and treatment.

Ayurvedic Institute
PO Box 23455, Albuquerque, NM 87192
(505) 291-9698

Bodytherapy Business Institute
4157 El Camino Way #C, Palo Alto, CA 94306
(415) 856-3151, (800) 888-1516 orders
Manual with information for bodyworkers about how to get reimbursed. Information about licensing for practitioners and consumers.

Cancer Control Society
2043 North Berendo, Los Angeles, CA 90027
(213) 663-7801
A non-profit educational, charitable, and scientific
society supported by contributions and memberships.

Coalition for Alternatives in Nutrition and Healthcare,
Inc. (CANAH)
PO Box B-12, Richlandtown, PA
(215) 346-8461

Council of Colleges of Acupuncture and Oriental
Medicine
1010 Wayne Avenue, Suite 1270,
Silver Spring, MD 20910
(301) 608-9175

Environmental Health Network
PO Box 1628, Harvey, LA
(504) 362-6574

Federation of Straight Chiropractic Organizations
642 Broad Street #9, Clifton, NJ 07013
(201) 777-1197, (800) 521-9856
Offers free referrals from 5,000 members who do
spinal adjustments, no supplemental therapies. All
are licensed doctors of chiropractic with over 5 years
of post-graduate training and internship through an
accredited chiropractic college.

Fetzer Institute
9292 West KL Avenue, Kalamazoo, MI 49009
(616) 375-2000

Holistic Dental Association
PO Box 5007, Durango, CO 81301
Offers referrals to 100 member dentists using
complementary methods. Written requests only, must
enclose self-addressed, stamped envelope. Referrals
are free, but a donation is requested.

Holistic Dental Association
974 North 21st Street, Newark, OH
(614) 366-3309

Holistic Health Association of the Princeton Area
(HHAPA)
Margie Herman, Pam Babbitt, David Nomitz
E-mail: mandala@lx.netcom.com
360 Nassau Street, Princeton, NJ
(609) 924-8580; Fax (609) 924-8711
Holistic Health Clearing house for New Jersey and
East Coast. Publishers of Holistic Living Magazine
and the Holistic Health Resource Directory.

Homeopathic Academy of Naturopathic Physicians
Susan Wolfer
E-mail: hanp@igc.apc.org (Web page: Web Page
http://www.healthy.net/HANP)
12132 Southeast Foster Place, Portland, OR 97266
(503) 761-3298; Fax (503) 762-1929
As a specialty society of the American Association of
Naturopathic Physicians (AANP), we certify
naturopathic doctors in homeopathy. Our directory is
available to the public, as well as our journal
Simillimum, and our annual case conference of cured
cases every November.

Human Ecology Action League (HEAL)
Katherine Collier
E-mail: HEALNatnl@aol.com
PO Box 29629, Atlanta, GA 30359-1126
(404) 248-1898; Fax (404) 248-0162
A national, nonprofit, education and information
organization founded in 1977 by physicians and
citizens concerned about the health effects of
environment exposures. HEAL offers publications and
regional support services provided by volunteers.

Institute for the Advancement of Health
16 East 53rd Street, Dept.D8, New York, NY
(212) 832-8282

International Academy of Holistic Health & Medicine
218 Avenue B, Redondo Beach, CA
(213) 540-0564

International Association of Holistic Health Practitioners
3419 Thom Boulevard, Las Vegas, NV
(702) 873-4542

International Chiropractors Association
1110 North Glebe Road, Suite 1000, Arlington, VA
(800) 423-4469

International College of Applied Kinesiology
(913) 542-1801
They will provide referrals for chiropractors.

International Foundation for Homeopathy
2366 Eastlake Avenue East, Suite 301, Seattle, WA
(206) 324-8230

International Foundation of Oriental Medicine
42062 Kissena Boulevard, Flushing, NY
(718) 321-8642

International Holistic Center, Inc.
PO Box 15103, Phoenix, AZ
(609) 957-3322

International Institute of Reflexology
E-mail: ftreflex@concentric.net
PO Box 12642, St. Petersburg, FL 33733-2642
(813) 348-4811; Fax (813) 381-2807
Promotes Foot Reflexology through a world-wide
referral service, training seminars offered
internationally, certification programs, and sales of
books, charts, reflexology foot aids.

International Society for the Study of Subtle Energies and
   Energy Medicine
   356 Goldco Circle, Golden, CO
   (303) 278-2228

Jin Shin Do Foundation of Bodymind Acupressure
   366 California Avenue, Suite 16, Palo Alto, CA
   (415) 328-1811

Lupus Acupuncture Network, Inc.
   PO Box 14332, Albuquerque, NM
   (505) 292-4722

National Acupuncture and Oriental Medicine Alliance
   14637 Starr Road Southeast, Olalla, WA 98359
   (206) 851-6896

National Acupuncture Detoxification Association
   PO Box 1927, Vancouver, WA 98668
   (360) 260-8620

National Association for Holistic Aromatherapy
   E-mail: info@naha.org
   PO Box 17622, Boulder, CO 80308
   (888) ASK-NAHA (275-6242),(314) 963-2071;
   Fax (314) 963-4454
   NAHA is an educational, non-profit organization
   dedicated to elevating the standards of aromatherapy
   education and practice. NAHA provides an exciting
   exchange of information through the quarterly journal
   Scentsitivity, International Conferences and Trade
   Shows, World of Aromatherapy book, and regional
   meetings across the U.S. and in parts of Canada. A
   directory of practitioners comes with membership.

National Association of Childbearing Centers (NACC)
   Kate Bauer
   E-mail: birthcenters.org
   3123 Gottschall Road, Perkiomenville, PA 18074
   (215) 234-8068; Fax (215) 234-8829
   The nation's most comprehensive resource on birth

centers. Working on public and policy levels in government, industry and the health professions, NACC is dedicated to developing quality, holistic services for childbearing families that promote self-reliance and confidence in birth and parenting.

National Center for Homeopathy
801 North Fairfax Street, Suite 306, Alexandria, VA
(703) 548-7790
They have a national registry to help you find a reputable homeopath in your area.

National Certification Commission for Acupuncture and Oriental Medicine
Cherlihy2@compuserve.com
1424 16th Street Northwest, Suite 105,
Washington, DC 20036
(202) 232-1404; Fax (202) 462-6157
Offers national certification programs in acupuncture, chinese herbology and oriental bodywork therapy.

National Council of Acupuncture Schools and Colleges
PO Box 954, Columbia, MD
(301) 997-4888

National Hospice Organization
1901 North Moor Street, Suite 901, Arlington, VA
(703) 243-5900

National Institute for the Clinical Application of Behavioral Medicine
PO Box 523, Mansfield Center, CT
(203) 429-2238

National Wellness Coalition
PO Box 3778, Washington, DC
(202) 872-5217; (202)333-1638

Nurse Healers - Professional Associates, Inc.
E-mail: nhpa@nursecominc.com
1211 Locust Street, Philadelphia, PA 19107
(215) 545-8079; Fax (215) 545-8107
NH-PA is an international network of members
interested in healing. NH-PA facilitates the exchange
of research findings, teaching strategies, and new
developments in the area of healing, and serves as the
principle clearinghouse for information on the
Krieger/Kunz model of Therapeutic Touch.

Pacific Institute of Aromatherapy
PO Box 6842, San Rafael, CA 94903
(415) 479-9121

People's Medical Society
462 Walnut Street, Allentown, PA
(215) 770-1670

Public Citizen Health Research Group
2000 P Street Northwest, Washington, DC
(202) 872-0320

Rosenthal Center for Alternative/Complementary
Medicine
College of P & S, Columbia University,
630 West 168th Street, New York, NY 10032
(212) 305-4755

Traditional Acupuncture Institute
American City Building, 10227 Wincopin Circle,
Suite 100, Columbia, MD 21044
(301) 596-6006

Whole Health Institute
4817 North County Road 29, Loveland, CO
(303) 679-4306

Research Organizations/Services

Alternative Medicine Information Line
(900) 443-4560, ext. 100 ($1.99 per minute)
Pre-recorded information gives the latest holistic
treatments and self-help tips for over 100 common
health problems.

American Health Federation
One Dana Road, Valhalla, NY
(914) 592-2600

Beth Israel Hospital/Department of Medicine
330 Brookline Avenue, LY-314, Boston, MA
(617) 667-3995

Best Doctors in America
129 First Avenue Southwest, Aiken, SC, 29801
(803) 648-0300; Fax (803) 641-1709
A reference book and service for finding the best
doctors in the U.S. resulting from a peer review-based
evaluation of more than ten thousand physicians.

Center for Complementary and Alternative Medicine
Research in Asthma, Allergy, and Immunology
University of California, Davis
Dr. Robert Hackman
E-mail: rmhackman@ucdavis.edu
Department of Nutrition, UC Davis, CA 95616
(916) 752-6575; Fax (916) 752-1297
Conduct scientific research into promising areas of
complementary/alternative medicine for asthma,
allergy, and immunology.

Center for Health Promotion Research & Development
University of Texas - Houston, PO Box 20186,
Houston, TX
(713) 792-8547

Center for Research on Complementary & Alternative
Therapies in Aging
Stanford University, 730 Welch Road, Palo Alto, CA
(415) 725-5012

Health Education Resources and Medical Extracts Service
(HERMES)
E-mail: sanfrancisco@sivananda.org
1200 Arguello Blvd., San Francisco, CA 94122
(415) 289-6550
Consumer medical search service that provides
medical information to both consumers and health
care practitioners. Special background in overseas
research, alternative and women's therapies.

The Health Resource, Inc.
E-mail: moreinfo@thehealthresource.com
564 Locust Avenue, Conway, AR 72032
(800) 949-0090, (501) 329-5272; Fax (501) 329-9489
Established in 1984, The Health Resource, Inc., is an
internationally acclaimed medical information service
that provides clients with individualized, bound
reports on their specific medical condition.
Information is included on the latest mainstream,
experimental, and alternative treatment options; plus
specialists, self-help tips, support groups, Internet
resources and a glossary. Reports are ready for
shipment in 3-5 business days and carry a 30-day,
money back guarantee.

Institute for Health and Healing
California Pacific Medical Center, PO Box 7999,
San Francisco, CA 94120
(415) 561-1374; Fax (415) 885-1561

Institute for Noetic Sciences
475 Gate Five Road, Suite 300, Sausalito, CA
(415) 331-5650

Kessler Institute for Rehabilitation
1199 Pleasant Valley Way, West Orange, NJ
(201) 243-6972

MEDLARS Management Section/National Library of
Medicine
8600 Rockville Place, Bethesda, MD
(800) 638-8480

Office of Alternative Medicine
6120 Executive Boulevard, Suite 450 (or National
Institutes of Health, 9000 Rockville Pike, Building 31,
Room 5B-38) Bethesda, Maryland 20892
(800) 531-1794, (301) 402-2466; Fax (301) 402-4741
OAM, which is within the National Institute of
Health, was created in 1992 to scientifically investigate
complementary and alternative therapies.
FAX Board: 301-402-2466 They have a "fax board", a
number you can phone and they will fax you
information.

Planetree Health Resource Center
450 Pacific Ave., Suite 250, San Francisco, CA 94133
(415) 923-3681; Fax (415) 673-2629
Nonprofit health and medical library, bookstore and
information service that provides access to a broad
range of conventional and alternative health
information.

Preventive Medicine Research Institute
900 Bridgeway, Suite 2, Sausalito, CA 94965
(415) 332-2525, (800) 775-7674; Fax (415) 332-5730
Founded by Dean Ornish, MD. The Institute is
involved with heart-health programs in hospitals and
will provide a list of recommended preventive care
practitioners.

Richard & Hinda Rosenthal Center for
Alternative/Complementary Medicine
Columbia University, College of Physicians & Surgeons.
    Fredi Kronenberg, Ph.D.
    630 West 168th Street, New York, NY 10032
    (212) 305-4755; Fax (212) 305-1495
    Has compiled a list of U.S. Medical Schools offering
    courses in Alternative Medicine.

Sharp Institute for Human Potential and Mind Body
Medicine
    The Holmes Center for Research in Holistic Healing
    600 South New Hampshire Avenue, Los Angeles, CA
    (213) 380-6176

University of Maryland
    Division of Complementary Medicine
    3rd Floor, Kernan Mansion, J.L. Kernan Hospital
    2200 North Forest Park Avenue, Baltimore, MD
    (410) 448-6871

University of Washington
    Health Policy Analysts Program
    (800) 989-8255

University of Virginia School of Nursing
    McLeod Hall, 15th and Lane Streets,
    Charlottesville, VA
    (804) 924-2744

World Research Foundation
    (818) 907-5483

Educational Organizations/Programs

Acupressure Institute of America
1533 Shatuck Avenue, Berkeley, CA 94709
(510) 845-1059

Barbara Brennan School of Healing
Internet: www.barbarabrennan.com
E-mail: bbshoffice@barbarabrennan.com
PO Box 2005, East Hampton, NY 11937
(516) 329-0951
Offers free referrals to healers who are graduates of a
four year certification program in healing the human
energy field. Request their International Directory of
Healers.

Cancer Control Society
Lorraine Rosenthal
2043 North Berendo Street, Los Angeles, CA 90027
(213) 663-7801
Information on Alternative Therapies and Nutritional
approach to Cancer and other diseases. Cancer
Control Society is a non-profit organization devoted to
educating the public on the prevention and control of
cancer and other diseases through nutrition, tests, and
other non-toxic alternative therapies. The Society also
offers help for other diseases such as Arthritis,
Diabetes, MS, and Heart Disease. Prevention is
stressed through eating natural foods, taking
supplements, minimizing stress, getting exercise and
natural light (full spectrum). An information packet,
which contains a doctor list, patient list, book list, diet
sheet, and prevention literature, is available upon
receipt of a $10.00 donation.

Chicago National College of Naprapathy
3330 North Milwaukee Avenue, Chicago, IL
(312) 282-2686

Clayton College of Natural Health
  2140 11th Avenue South, Suite 305,
  Birmingham, AL 35205
  (800) 995-4590, (205) 933-2215
  College of Natural Health, Nutrition, and Holistic
  Lifestyles.

College of Ayur-Veda Health Center
  PO Box 282, Fairfield, IA 52556
  (515) 472-8477

Common Ground
  920 North Franklin Street, Suite 301, Chicago, IL
  (847) 940-7870

Deepak Chopra Seminars
  Nora Kinsella
  E-mail: quantpub@aol.com
  7630 Fay Avenue, La Jolla, CA 92037
  (800) 757-8897; Fax (508) 440-8411
Journey to the Boundless
  A weekend seminar on self-healing where you will
  learn the ancient healing power of Ayurvedic
  medicine, determine your dosha (mind-body type)
  and the best lifestyle for you; discover how to reverse
  the biological markers of aging and maintain your
  youthfulness; and create the spontaneous fulfillment
  of your desires and reach higher states of
  consciousness.
Seduction of the Spirit
  An ideal opportunity for you to explore your own
  spirituality, as well as restore the harmony within and
  tap into your body's inner intelligence. It is highly
  recommended if you are ready to delve deeper into
  your spiritual development and seek personal growth
  and transformation.
Training in Mind-Body Medicine
  In this intensive program, you will explore natural

and holistic approaches to health. Learn to use mind-body insights, techniques for both disease prevention and as a complement to the traditional Western treatment of disease. You will delve into the exciting new information on the potential healing relationship between mind and body. Your ideas and inspiration can be shared with other interested health care professionals.

Health Care Futures
  Mary Ann Neis, RN, M.N.
  and Barbara Manley-Wheeler, RN, M.S.
  E-mail: neisma@aol.com
  c/o Mary Ann Neis, 370 Rosecrans Street, #301, San Diego, CA 92106
  (619) 225-9955
  Provides workshops, consultation, and lectures on topics such as: A general overview of complementary/alternative medicine; Descriptions of Complementary Modalities; and Stress-Reduction Techniques for Use at Work and Home; and Leaders in the Complementary Medicine field, with discussion about their areas of interest. The workshops are informational, experiential, and tailor-made to the organization or group. They can be 1 hour, three hours, half or whole days, or a weekend seminar. The workshops are conceived around your specific needs and are valuable for anyone with an interest in restoring balance, awakening their heart, or reducing stress in their lives. Seminars for health care workers are designed to educate about alternative therapies dealing with prevention and treatment of chronic disease processes.

Health Horizons
  PO Box 278205, Sacramento, CA
  (800) 769-9355

Himalayan Institute of Glenview
    1505 Greenwood Road, Glenview, IL
    (847) 724-0300

Hollyhock
    PO Box 127, Manson's Landing,
    Cortes Island CANADA, BC
    (800) 933-6339

International Foundation of Bio-Magnetics
    5447 East 5th Street, Suite 111, Tucson, AZ 85711
    (520) 323-7951
    Offers free referrals to 60 practitioners of Bio-Magnetic
    Touch Healing(, a simple, light touch healing
    technique. All have completed the Introductory Class
    and many have completed the Certification Program.

International School of Shiatsu
    Amy Harris
    10 South Clinton Street, Suite 300, Doylestown, PA
    (215) 340-9918

John F. Kennedy University
    Graduate School for Holistic Studies
    E-mail: HOLISTIC@jfku.edu
    12 Altarinda Road, Orinda, CA 94563
    (510) 254-0105; Fax (510)254-3322
    One of the first accredited academic programs in the
    nation devoted to the integration of body, mind and
    spirit.

Landmark Education Corporation
    Corporate Office (415) 981-8850; Fax (415)616-2411
    Top-notch programs relating to personal
    transformation and breakthrough thinking.

Mind/Body Medical Clinic
Harvard Medical School
E-mail: mbclinic@west.bidmc.harvard.edu
Beth Israel Deaconess Medical Center,
One Deaconess Road, West Campus
Boston, MA 02215
(617) 632-9530; Fax (617) 632-7383
Outpatient medical clinic designed to help those with chronic illness or stress related symptoms better manage their conditions. Ten to 13 week programs for general stress-related symptoms, cancer, cardiac rehab., cardiac risk reduction, chronic pain, HIV+/AIDS, infertility, insomnia, and menopause.

National Wellness Institute, Inc.
1045 Clark Street, Suite 210, Stevens Point, WI
(800) 243-8694

Omega Institute for Holistic Studies
260 Lake Drive, Rhinebeck, NY
(914) 266-4444

Practical Application of Intimate Relationship Skills (PAIRS)
3705 South George Mason Drive, Suite C3S, Falls Church, VA 22041
(800) 842-7470
For learning about yourself and your behavior with respect to intimate relationships. The program is based on the work of Virginia Satir.

Silva Method
(800) 745-8262, (630) 761-1463
Teaches how to use more of the brain and mind to help you get more of what is you want - better health, more happiness, more success.

Society for the Universal Human/Living Enrichment
Center
29500 Southwest Grahams Ferry Road,
Wilsonville, OR
(800) 893-1000

Western Michigan University
Graduate Certificate Program in Holistic Health Care
Molly B. Vass, Ed.D and Brenda Bell
web site under construction:
http://141.218.1.101/hhs/htm/hh.htm
College of Health and Human Services,
Kalamazoo, MI 49008-5174
(616) 387-3800; Fax (616) 387-3348

Health Insurance

Aetna U.S. Health
(800) 872-3862
Covers acupuncture, chiropractic, nutrition
counseling.

Allina Health System
(612) 992-2000
Medical Health Plan wellness program covers
acupressure, acupuncture, and chiropractic in
Minnesota, North Dakota, South Dakota, and
Wisconsin.

Alternative Health Benefits Services/Alliance for
Alternatives in Healthcare, Inc.
PO Box 6279, Thousand Oaks, CA 91359
(800) 966-8467, (805) 494-7818; Fax (805) 494-8528
Insurance for alternative and conventional treatments.

Alternative Health Plan
(800) 374-6003
Insurance for alternative and conventional treatments.

American Medical Security
(800) 232-5432
HealthCare Choices plan covers a range of
alternatives in Arizona.

American National
(800) 899-6803
Covers a range of alternatives.

American Western Life Insurance Company
(800) 925-5323
Wellness plans cover a range of alternatives in 6
Western states.

AmeriHealth
(800) 454-7651
Covers chiropractic and mental wellness program for
drinking cessation in 7 states.

Bienstar
(888) 692-4363
Covers acupuncture, chiropractic, nutrition, and counseling in New York.

Blue Cross of California
(818) 703-2345
Covers a range of alternatives in California.

Blue Cross/Blue Shield of South Carolina
(803) 788-0222
Covers the Dean Ornish program in South Carolina.

Blue Cross of Washington and Alaska
(800) 752-6663
Have holistic-care packages, which covers the care of acupuncturists, homeopaths, and naturopaths.

CIGNA HealthCare
Call (800) information for the number in your State.
Covers a range of alternatives.

Co-op America
(800) 584-7336
Covers chiropractic care.

Family Health Plan
(419) 241-6501
Covers chiropractic care, nutrition counseling, and physical therapy in Ohio and Michigan.

Fortis Benefits
(800) 955-1586
Covers a range of alternatives.

Great West Life Assurance
(800) 537-2033, ext. 4200
Covers a range of alternatives.

Guardian Life
(800) 662-1006
Covers naturopathy.

Harvard Community Health Plan
(800) 543-7429
Gives discounts on Personal Health Improvement Program for stress-related illness, chronic disease, mood disorders in Massachusetts.

Harvard Pilgrim Health Care
(888) 333-4742
Covers chiropractic and nutrition counseling in Massachusetts and Rhode Island.

HealthPartners Health Plans
Phoenix, AZ
(800) 351-1505
Covers alternative services offered at the Arizona Center for Health and Medicine.

John Alden Life
(800) 435-7969
Covers acupuncture and chiropractic.

Kaiser Permanente
(800) 464-4000
Covers a range of alternatives.

Mutual of Omaha
(800) 456-0228
Covers acupuncture, naturopathy, and Dean Ornish program.

National Insurance Consumer Helpline
(800) 942-4242
Provides general help with choosing an agent or insurer.

New England Mutual Life
(800) 237-4878
Covers acupressure, acupuncture, chiropractic.

New York Life
(800) 338-8113, (718) 899-3600
Covers a range of alternatives in New York and Connecticut.

Oxford HMO
(800) 844-6222
Offers the nation's first credentialed network of alternative care practitioners, including acupuncturists, chiropractors, massage therapists, and nutritionists. Currently only available in New York and New Jersey.

Pacific Mutual Life
(800) 733-7020
Covers naturopathy.

Physicians Health Service
(800) 441-5741
Covers naturopathy and acupuncture.

Phoenix Home Life/Phoenix American Life
(800) 343-0944
Covers a range of alternatives.

Principal Mutual
(800) 986-3343
Covers a range of alternatives.

Prudential
(800) 346-3778
Covers a range of alternatives.

Sentry Life
(800) 533-7827
Covers acupressure, biofeedback, lifestyle counseling; available in most states.

Suburban Health Plan
(203) 734-4466
Covers a range of alternatives.

TrueCare, Inc.
(708) 660-9156
A network of holistic, alternative, and complementary care practitioners in the Chicago area. Members receive discounted services.

Trustmark
(800) 366-6663, (800) 347-0889
Covers aromatherapy and chiropractic and is
available in most states.

Tufts Total Health Plan
(800) 462-0224
Covers nutrition counseling and stress management
in Massachusetts, Maine, New Hampshire, and
Rhode Island.

UniCare
(617) 572-7327
Covers biofeedback and chiropractic; if administered
by an MD also covers acupressure, acupuncture, and
naturopathy.

Woodmen Accident and Life
(800) 869-0355
Covers chemical dependency counseling, chiropractic,
counseling for mental disorders in most states.

World
(800) 600-7760, ext. 3367
Covers naturopathy.

Publications: Articles, Books, Studies

* *Books which I Consider Excellent Resources*
** *Books which I Consider Especially Excellent Resources*

A Consumer's Guide to Alternative Health Care.
Craig Clayton and Virginia McCullough.
Adams Publishing, 1995.
Describes a range of alternative therapies.

Alternative Health Care Resources.
Brett Jason Sinclair. Parker Publishing Company, 1992.
Provides information about self-help groups,
professional organizations, institutions, foundations,
journals, magazines, and newsletters that provide
information on alternative treatments, disease-
preventive lifestyle changes, and health-related issues.
A handy resource, slightly outdated.

Alternative Medicine: The Definitive Guide.
An extensive reference guide. Although it appears to
be extremely comprehensive, I found it hard to use
(it seemed overwhelming).

* *Alternative Medicine: What Works.*
'A comprehensive, easy-to-read review of the scientific
evidence, pro and con.' This book explains all those
studies that have been done in language that is easily
understood. The tone is friendly and the work is
extensively referenced.

Alternative Medicine Yellow Pages.
Provides good background about alternative medicine
and how to select an alternative practitioner. List
alternative therapies and therapists as well as some
products by type of therapy and location.

American Holistic Health Association Complete Guide to Alternative Medicine.
> William Collinge, MPH, Ph.D. Warner Books, 1996.
> An easy to read introduction to some options in alternative medicine.

Choices in Healing: Integrating the Best of Conventional and Complementary Approaches to Cancer.
> Michael Lerner. MIT Press, 1994.

8 Weeks to Optimum Health.
> Andrew Weil, MD.
> A multi-faceted approach to healing yourself, presented in language that is easy to understand.

** *Encyclopedia of Alternative Medicine.*
> A beautiful, stunning, portrayal of various alternative therapies. A useful, and fun, reference.

Everything You Always Wanted to Know About Energy But Were Too Tired to Ask.
> Dr. Paul Varnas and Barbara J. Stepp, CH, 1996.
> A practical, enjoyable and motivational book about how to have better health and more energy.

* *Five Steps to Selecting the Best Alternative Medicine: A Guide to Complementary and Integrative Health Care,*
> Mary and Michael Morton. New World Library, 1996.
> This book provides a lot of information for understanding and using alternative medicine. I was impressed by how comprehensive it is. I found it hard to read, but I would definitely recommend it as a handy reference.

Health Care Choices for Today's Consumer.
> Edited by Marc S. Miller. Living Planet Press, 1995.
> While not focused on alternative medicine, this book covers the basics very well, and in easy to understand language. They also publish companion guides for

Chicago, San Francisco, Seattle-Tacoma, Washington, DC, and Boston. Health Care Choices for Today's Consumer is "a step-by-step sourcebook for: choosing the best health plan for your family; saving money on everyday care; evaluating doctors, specialists, and hospitals; finding health care services for women, children, and seniors".

Healing With Love.
Leonard Laskow, MD. Harper/SanFrancisco, 1992.
Very interesting research with actions you can take to use energy in your own healing.

Manifesto for a New Medicine.
James S. Gordon, MD, 1996.
An easy to read, inspiring book about the possibilities of integrated health care.

Medical Advisor: The Complete Guide to Alternative and Conventional Treatments.
Time/Life Books, 1996.
A very thorough, and somewhat overwhelming resource.

** *Mind Body Medicine: How to Use Your Mind for Better Health.*
Consumer Reports Books.
Edited by Daniel Goleman, Ph.D. and Joel Gurin, 1996.
An excellent resource, very empowering, with chapters contributed by well known experts covering: mind/body basics, the mind's role in illness, what you can do, and becoming an active patient. Very well referenced, with resources for further inquiries.

New Choices in Natural Healing.
Edited by Bill Gottlieb, Editor-in Chief, Prevention Magazine Health Books. Rodale Press, Inc.
"Over 1,800 of the Best Self-Help Remedies from the World of Alternative Medicine."

Reclaiming our Health: Exploding the Medical Myth and Embracing the Source of True Healing.
John Robbins. HJ Kramer, 1996.
A very interesting, very readable book about the health field. Full of factual information, yet easy to follow.

Your Body Believes Every Word You Say: The Language of the Body/Mind Connection
Barbara Hoberman Levine. Aslan Publishing, 1991.
Shows us how our language can sabotage our wellness and how we can use illness as a tool for increased self-understanding and healing.

Your Personal Net Doctor: Your Guide to Health and Medical Advice on the Internet and Online Services.
Wolff New Media, 1996.
A great resource that makes using the Web easy.

Journals

Alternative Therapies in Health and Medicine
101 Columbia, Aliso Viejo, CA
(800) 899-1712

Alternative Therapies
Subscription Information: (800) 345-8112
Alternative Therapies is a forum for the development of and sharing information concerning the practical use of alternative therapies in preventing and treating disease, healing illness, and promoting health. Alternative Therapies does not endorse any particular methodology, but promotes the evaluation and appropriate use of all effective approaches from the physical to the transpersonal. The Journal publishes a variety of disciplined inquiry methods, including high-quality scientific research. The Journal encourages the integration of alternative-therapies

with conventional medical practice in a way that provides for a rational, individualized, comprehensive approach to healthcare.

Arlin J. Brown Information Center, Inc.
PO Box 251, Fort Belvoir, VA
(703) 451-8638

Bestways Magazine, Inc.
PO Box 570, Oak Park, IL
(312) 848-8100

New Age Journal/Holistic Health Directory
42 Pleasant Street, Watertown, MA
(617) 926-0200

Web Sites

Recommended Sites

Alternative Medicine: Health Care Information Resources
http://wwwhsl.mcmaster.ca/tomflem/altmed.html
Lots of links, and descriptions of the links!

Alternative Medicine - HealthWorld Online
http://www.healthy.net/index.html
Many interesting links, easy to use.
http://www.healthy.net/clinic/therapy/integrating.htm
Interesting articles about the integration of Alternative
and Mainstream Medicine.

Alternative Medicine Home Page
http://www.pitt.edu/~cbw/altm.html
Easy to use, good place to start. Lots of links! "This
page is a jumpstation for sources of information on
unconventional, unorthodox, unproven, or alternative,
complementary, innovative, integrative therapies."
http://www.pitt.edu/~cbw/refe.html
Studies on use of Alternative Therapies.
http://www.pitt.edu/~cbw/oam.html
Complete information about the Office of Alternative
Medicine and OAM Alternative Medicine Centers.
The 1992 Congressional mandate establishing OAM
stated that the purpose is to "facilitate the evaluation
of alternative medical treatment modalities" for the
purpose of determining their effectiveness and to help
integrate treatments into mainstream medical practice.
The OAM does not serve as a referral agency for
various alternative medicine treatment modalities or
individual practitioners.

American Holistic Health Association
http://www.healthy.net/ahha/
Lots of information and links about holistic health.

General Complementary Medicine References
http://www.forthrt.com/~chronicl/archiv.htm
Lots of links, little additional information. Also has information about discussion groups and mailing lists.

Healthy Solutions
www.healthy-solutions-us.com
Updated information about the book *Where to go When You're Hurting: A Healing Resource Guide.*

New York Online Access to Health (NOAH)
http://www.noah.cuny.edu/alternative/alternative.html
Links organized by "integrated" healing approach.

Yahoo! - Health: Alternative Medicine
http://www.yahoo.com/health/alternative_medicine
Loads of links. Easy to use. Plan on spending a lot of time here. Great place to start your search.

Other Sites

Alchemical Medicine Research and Teaching Association Home Page
http://www.teleport.com/~amrta/
Links to related information. Names and addresses for medical and health organizations and associations.

AltHealth Search
http://www.althealthsearch.com/
"A resource center designed to help you, the visitor, find alternative medical practitioners in your area. AltHealth Search has over 173,000 listings of

alternative health care practitioners throughout the United States." Information about Certifications and Abbreviations, State and National and Accreditation Agencies.

ALTMED Home Page
http://www.teleport.com/~mattlmt/
Provides a directory for finding registered practitioners world wide.

American Association of Alternative Healers
http://www.concentric.net/~Aaah/
May be fun to explore.

Ask Dr. Weil
http://www.drweil.com
A fun, informative, eclectic site hosted by Dr. Andrew Weil. Includes his 8 Weeks to Optimal Health. His Referrals page provides links to professional organizations.

Center for the Advancement of Health
http://www.cfah.org/
"The Center for the Advancement of Health was established to be a voice for change in the health system. The mission of the Center is to achieve the widespread acceptance and application of an expanded view of health that recognizes the role of behavioral, psychological, social, and environmental as well as physical factors in promoting health and preventing and treating disease." Links to related sites.

Center for the Study of Complementary and Alternative Therapies
http://www.med.Virginia.edu/nursing/centers/alt-ther.html
The Center for the Study of Complementary and Alternative Therapies (CSCAT) is a NIH-funded center established as a mechanism to stimulate research in complementary and alternative medicine (CAM) therapies.

Complementary and Alternative Medicine Program and
Stanford (CAMPS)
> http://scrdp.stanford.edu/camps.html
>> Information about research, and related resources.
>> Links to OAM Complementary and Alternative
>> Medicine Research Sites.

Comprehensive Health and Wellness for mind/body/spirit
> http://www.wholeliving.com/
>> Looks like there is a lot of activity, may be fun to
>> explore.

Dr. Bower's Alternative & Complementary Medicine Home
Page
> http://galen.med.virginia.edu/~pjb3s/ComplementaryHomePage.html
>> Presented by The Dogwood Institute, a non-profit
>> corporation. Information and links.

HealthGate
> http://www.healthgate.com/
>> "Your online source for health, wellness, and
>> biomedical information"

Holistic America, Inc.
> http://www.planetwellness.com/holisticamerica/
>> Articles and information about holistic happenings.

Holistic Internet Community
> http://www.holistic.com/
>> "The Holistic Internet Community (HIC) is here to
>> provide a place for everyone
>> to exchange information and congregate to promote a
>> healing understanding of our relationships to each
>> other, the world and the cosmos. This is a place for
>> you to locate the resources and tools to live a balanced
>> life, and to find support during the difficult times
>> along the way. As the Holistic Internet Community
>> grows, its direction will be guided by your
>> comments."

Institute for Holistic Healing Studies
www.healthy.net/HANP

Institute for Holistic Healing Studies
http://userwww.sfsu.edu/~jasonb/holistic.htm
San Francisco State University. Links to other Holistic
Health Sites.

MedAccess
http://www.medaccess.com/
Although not particularly holistic, good source of
health and medical information. Lists thousands of
physicians and hospitals.

MedWeb: Biomedical Internet Resources
http://www.gen.emory.edu/MEDWEB/medweb.html

Section II: Healing Institutions

Listings by State

Foxhollow Wellness Spa, 179
Institute for Mind Body Medicine, 162
Marino Center for Progressive Health, 163
Reiki Training Institute, 166
University of Massachusetts Medical Center
    Stress Reduction Clinic, 177
Maharishi Ayur-Veda Health Center, 180

Michigan
Creative Health Institute: Living Food Lifestyle, 156
Creative Wellness, 156
Earth Community Center, 157
Synthesis Center, 168

Minnesota
Health Recovery Center, 160
Preventive Medicine Associates, 166

Missouri
Shealy Institute, 167
Surfside Chiropractic, 168

Montana
Blue: A Center for Life, 152
Natural Medicine Clinic, 164

Nebraska
Alegent Health System, 171
    Bergan-Mercy Medical Center

Nevada
Ayurvedic Living Center, 151

New Hampshire
Genesis Alternative Health Center, 158

New Jersey
Amwell Health Center, 150
Bio-Preventive Medical Care, 151
Center for Natural Healing Arts, 155
Princeton Associates for Total Health, 166

Healing Clinics/Centers

A Sante Health Center
455 Los Gatos Boulevard, Suite 107, Los Gatos, CA
(408) 358-2188

Acupuncture and Healing Therapies
Maxine M. Shapiro
E-mail: gns@world.std.com
53 Marshall Street, Newton, MA 02159
(617) 965-5251; Fax (617) 964-3509
Maxine M. Shapiro, nationally certified in
acupuncture and massage, "Holistic Health Detective"
uses nutrition, homeopathy, Chinese herbs, energetic
cranial-sacral work, and Feng Shui.

Agape Fellowship Center
Shirley Saylors-Clarkson, RN
3017 North Causeway Boulevard, Suite C,
Metairie, LA 70002
(504) 831-1006
Holistic massage therapy, colonic irrigation with
nutritional guidance, foot reflexology, integration
counseling, cotyledon, music therapy.

Alaska Alternative Medicine Center
3201 C Street, Suite 306, Anchorage, AK
(907) 561-4933

Alaska Massage Center
851 Westpoint #201, Wasilla, AK
(907) 373-7117

Alternative Medicine Clinic
Frank Yurasek, MA, Ac.T.
8 South Michigan Avenue, Suite 1418,
Chicago, IL 60603
(312) 456-3000; Fax (312) 456-3045
Acupuncture, Homeopathy, Herbology, Oriental
Bodywork, Chiropractic, Western Medicine, T'ai
Qi/Qi Gung.

Alternative Health Partners
Dion Richetti, D.C.
E-mail: AAHP@aol.com
4753 North Broadway, Suite 1126, Chicago, IL 60640
(773) 561-3400; Fax (773) 561-8225

Alternative Medicine Clinic
15611 Bel-Red Road, Bellevue, WA
(206) 881-2224

American Holistic Center, Arizona
Steve Borst
(703) 453-6899

American Metabolic Institute
www.ami-health.com
555 Saturn Boulevard, M/S 432, San Diego, CA 92154
(619) 267-1107; Fax (619) 267-1109

American Whole Health - Lincoln Park Center
Keith Berndtson, MD or David Edelberg, MD
990 West Fullerton #300, Chicago, IL 60614
(773) 296-6700; Fax (773) 296-1131
One of America's largest centers of physician
supervised alternative medicine with five board
certified physicians and twenty practitioners from a
variety of complementary therapies. These include
herbal medicine, chiropractic, nutrition, naprapathy,
traditional Chinese medicine, Reiki, homeopathy,
massage therapy, psychoneuroimmunology and
counseling. Physicians are on the staffs of Rush-
Presbyterian, Illinois Masonic, Grant and Columbus
Hospitals. Many services are covered by conventional
insurance programs.

Amwell Health Center
450 Amwell Road, Suite E, Belle Mead, NJ
(908) 359-1775

Arbor Vitae Chiropractic
Paul G. Varnas, D.C., D.A.B.C.N., C.C.N.
3056 North Sheffield, Chicago, IL 60657
(773) 525-0007
Specializing in Applied Kinesiology.

Associates In Family Health Care
4 Broadway, Valhalla, NY
(914) 681-5112

Ayurvedic Living Center
Beverlee Cannon
8429 Stapleton, Las Vegas, NV 89128
(702) 363-1585; Fax (702) 255-4322
Full service, mind/body/spirit holistic health center.
Naturopathic doctor, ayurvedic pulse practitioner,
panchakarma therapies, yoga and yogic breathing
instruction, meditation training and group practice,
herbs, teas, churnas, oil and tinctures, books. Cooking
classes, workshops and retreats.

Balancing Center
1871 North Clybourn, Chicago, IL 60614
(312) 327-3333

Bio Preventive Medical Care
235 Prospect Avenue, Hackensack, NJ
(201) 525-1155

Biscayne Institutes of Health and Living, Inc.
Mark DiCowden, Administrator
E-mail: bri@gate.net
2785 Northeast 183rd Street, Aventura, FL 33160
(800) 454-3348, (305) 932-8994; Fax (305) 932-9362
A comprehensive rehabilitation center specializing in
Brain Injury, Spinal Cord Injury, Amputations, and
Chronic Disease, incorporating mind and body
healing. Wellness and prevention programs also
available for general healthcare. Treating Pediatrics to
Geriatrics. A healthcare community.

Block, Keith, MD
Medical Director or the Cancer Treatment Program
and Medical Chief of Nutritional and Behavioral
*Oncology at the **Edgewater Medical Center***
899 Sherman Avenue, Suite 515, Evanston, IL 60201
(708) 492-3040
Dr. Block is known for using conventional and holistic
approaches for treating cancer.

Blue: A Center for Life
Blue Sky Road, Lavina, MT
(406) 575-4346

BodyMind & Breath Center of Kauai
Joan Levy, MSW, ACSW, LCSW, LSW
E-mail: heal-hi@aloha.net (www.lauhala.com/joan)
PO Box 160, Kapaa, HI 96746
(800) 599-5488; Phone/Fax: (808) 822-5488;
Offering Mind Healing Intensives for individuals,
couples and small groups coming to Kauai interested
in swift, mindbody breakthrough and personal
empowerment. Breathwork, Deep Emotional Release,
Belief Restructuring, and Consciousness Training.

Healing Arts Resources Kauai
Phone/Fax: (808) 823-8088
A non-profit, professional association offering a free
information and referral service to over 70 holistic
practitioners on Kauai.

Cancer Treatment Centers of America
www.cancercenter.com
(800) 234-0497

Carolina Center for Alternative and Nutritional Medicine
Brooke Thompson
E-mail: center@he.net
4505 Fair Meadow Lane, Suite 111, Raleigh, NC 27607
(919)571-4391; Fax (919) 571-8968

Comprehensive, multi-dimensional treatment center using intravenous vitamin and mineral therapies, ozone, hydrogen peroxide, chelation, lymphatic massage, and colon hydrotherapy for thorough body cleansing and improvement in overall body metabolism. We work with chronic viral and bacterial infections, cardiovascular disorders, and all immune dysfunctions.

Center for the Healing Arts
325 Boston Post Road, Orange, CT 06477
(203) 799-7733
The integration of environmental medicine, allergy testing (by provocative neutralization), nutrition, biological dentistry, including mercury removal, chemical and heavy metal detoxification, pediatrics and family medicine, natural medicine, intravenous replacement of nutrients, psychological therapies, comprehensive weight control, rheumatology, neuraltherapy, and prolotherapy.

Center for Holistic Dentistry
Harold E. Ravins, DDS
12381 Wilshire Boulevard, Suite 103,
Los Angeles, CA 90025
(310) 207-4617

Center for Holistic Medicine
1251 Shermer Road, Northbrook, IL 60062
(708) 509-8903

Center for Integrated Health Care
Dr. Alan F. Bain
E-mail: cihc@net-cci.com
104 South Michigan Avenue, Suite 705,
Chicago, IL 60603
(312) 236-7010; Fax (312) 236-7190
Our approach to chronic illness is two-fold: Health management with traditional medical support

enfolded into the larger holistic framework of complementary health care. Services include: internal medicine, medical acupuncture, osteopathic and nutritional medicine, allergy elimination, and psychology referrals.

Center for Mind-Body Medicine
Paul Epstein ND
9 Berkeley Street, Norwalk, CT 06850
(203) 853-6800; Fax (203) 838-7510
Paul Epstein, ND, is a naturopathic physician. His approach views illness and symptoms as an opportunity for growth, transformation, and healing. He specializes in mind-body therapies of mindfulness meditation, guided imagery, relaxation, and stress management. He integrates mind-body medicine with clinical nutrition, dietary counseling, herbal and homeopathic medicine, to support and stimulate each person's process of self-healing.

Center for Mind-Body Medicine
James S. Gordon, MD, Director
E-mail: cmbm@idsonline.com
5225 Connecticut Avenue Northwest, Suite 414, Washington, DC 20015
(202) 966-7338; Fax (202) 966-2589
A non-profit, educational organization offering community outreach programs, monthly workshops, and mind-body skills groups to the local community and training programs to professionals nation-wide.

Center for Mind-Body Medicine: Professional Training Program
Carol Goldberg
cmbm@idsonline.com
5225 Connecticut Avenue Northwest, #414, Washington, DC 20015
(202) 966-7338; Fax (202) 966-2589

An experimental training program for health and mental health professionals in leading mind-body skills groups for optimal wellness and for people living with chronic illness.

Center for Natural Healing Arts
87 Midland Avenue, Montclair, NJ
(201) 744-0388

Center for Natural Healing Arts
61 North Maple Avenue, Ridgewood, NJ
(201) 445-8100

Center for Natural Medicine, Inc.
1330 Southeast 39th Avenue, Portland, OR
(503) 232-1100

Center for Pranic Restoration
1330 East High Street, Springfield, OH
(513) 324-4660

Center for Results
1119 13th Avenue, Altoona, PA
(814) 944-2290

Center for Traditional Acupuncture
American City Building, Suite 108, Columbia, MD
(301) 997-3770

Chopra Center for Well-Being
7630 Fay Avenue, La Jolla, CA 92037
(888) 424-6772; Fax (508)440-8411
The Center offers an integrated approach to mind-body medicine and Ayurveda. Individual treatments as well as comprehensive Ayurvedic programs over multiple days are offered. Our Ayurvedic staff, who are also Western trained physicians and nurses, will prescribe a series of specialized treatments to enhance the immune system, tone skin and muscles, loosen impurities, and address specific health concerns.

Primordial Sound Meditation (PSM) and Magic of Healing are taught at the Center and around the world by trained instructors. PSM uses an individually selected vibratory sound, or mantra, to create a quieting influence so that one can go beyond the daily activity of the mind into quieter and deeper levels of thinking. PSM reduces stress and fatigue, sharpens awareness, and soothes our entire being: body, mind and spirit. Magic of Healing teaches mind-body principles and techniques that one can use in every day life. This practical course will show that the mind creates the deepest influence on the body and that freedom from illness depends upon restoring the memory of wholeness in mind and body. Magical Beginnings, Enchanted Lives is a new pre-natal course for pregnant couples which combines the best of traditional medicine with groundbreaking information on pregnancy. This seven week course guides couples with all the practical information they need for a healthy pregnancy and delivery and teaches the miracle of bringing a new soul into the world.

Chrysalis Natural Medicine Center
1008 Milltown Road, Wilmington, DE
(302) 994-0565

Colorado Center for Healing Touch, Inc.
198 Union Boulevard, Suite 204, Lakewood, CO
(303) 989-0581

Creative Health Institute: Living Food Lifestyle
Matthew Evans
E-mail: christage@orion.branch-co.lib.mi.us
918 Union City Road, Union City, MI 49094
(517) 278-6260; Fax (517) 278-5837
We offer a hands on learning program based on the Living Foods Lifestyle developed by Dr. Ann Wigmore. We also offer therapeutic massage.

Creative Wellness
  2025 Abbott Road, East Lansing, MI
  (517) 351-9240

Center for Integrated Health Care
  104 South Michigan Avenue, Suite 705, Chicago, IL
  (312) 236-7010

Dana Mothercare: Supporting services for the childbearing year.
  70 West Erie, Chicago, IL 60610
  (312) 266-9241

Doctor's Center for Preventive Medicine
  159 West 53rd Street, New York, NY
  (212) 333-2626

Dogwood Institute
  2200 Old Ivey Road, PO Box 5752, Charlottesville, VA
  (804) 296-4160

Dorothy Harrison, RN
  3931 South Dakota Avenue Northeast,
  Washington, DC
  (202) 832-5477

Dr. Jansen's Wellness Center
  1275 Fall River Avenue (Route 6), Seekonk, MA
  (800) 520-8733

Earth Community Center
  116 Floral Avenue, Mount Clemens, MI
  (810) 463-3486

Essence Chiropractic Center
  Dr. Sue Brown
  25 West 330 Geneva Road, Carol Stream, IL 60188-2328
  (630) 690-6080
  At Essence Chiropractic Center, Dr. Sue Brown utilizes a system called Network Spinal Analysis (NSA). NSA initiates a process of removing interference in the

nervous system so as to promote healing by releasing the causes, not just treating the symptom. Many people who began care because of a specific symptom have stayed long after that symptom was gone because they felt other things changing within themselves as well. The Mission of the Center is to awaken each individual to their own internal wisdom, whether by touch, by word, or by community participation, thus releasing more vital energy into their system and improving the quality of their life.

Excellence Quest Institute
Barbara J. Stepp
222 Pearson East, Chicago, IL 60611
(312) 587-0440
Co-author of *Everything You Always Wanted to Know About Energy But Were too Tired to Ask* with Dr. Paul Varnas.

Europa Therapeutic Massage & Acupressure Clinic
455 South 300 East, Suite 103, Salt Lake City, UT
(801) 355-6300

Family Health, Sport, Financial, Intl.
5831 Kenneth Avenue, Fair Oaks, CA
(800) 373-9237

Family Practice Center
312 East Alta Vista, Ottumwa, IA
(515) 683-3101

Fitness Quest
1080 Main Street South, Suites 3 and 5, Woodbury, CT
(203) 263-4399

Future 5000 Massage Therapy Center
607 East Abram Street, Suite 16, Arlington, TX
(817) 548-9223

Genesis Alternative Health Center
Londonderry Square Suite 209A, Londonderry, NH
(603) 434-4113

Global Yoga and Wellness Center
Rhonda Kantor, RN, B.S.N., H.N.C. (Holistic
Nurse Certified)
1608 North Milwaukee Avenue, Suite 212,
Chicago, IL 60647
(773) 489-1510
The center offers a variety of programs and classes
applying the holistic approach toward health,
wellness and healing. The structure and philosophy
of the center encourages participants to choose from a
variety of paths toward continued wellness. We offer:
Yoga classes (Hatha, Pre-Natal, Kundalini, Iyengar,
and yoga for special needs), Massage, T'ai Chi, Belly
Dance, Mother/Baby Wellness and Parenting Group,
childbirth education, labor support (Doula), yoga
instructors workshops, women's groups, and
relaxation/stress reduction classes.

Healing Arts Center on the River (Ancilla Health Care)
Karen K. Dupuis
E-mail: kdupuis@ancilla.org
1625 East Jefferson Boulevard, Mishawaka, IN 46545
(219) 257-2295; Fax (219) 257-2298
Complementary Healing Modalities: Massage,
Acupuncture, Herbs, Reflexology, Energy Work, Art
Therapy, Transpersonal Counseling, Pastoral
Counseling, Stress Management, Nutrition Services,
Holistic Health Assessments, Flower Essences, Herbal
Body Wraps, Holistic Physician Consultations,
Metabolic Testing, Extensive Education Programs, T'ai
Chi, Yoga, Meditation, Vegetarian Cooking, Dream
Therapy Group, Healing Touch, Reiki, and Manual
Lymph Drainage.

Healing Arts Center
753 North Main Street, Cottonwood, AZ
(520) 634-7470

Healing Arts Center of Covina
642 South Eremland Drive, Covina, CA
(909) 598-6680

Health and Healing Clinic
2300 California Street, Suite 200,
San Francisco, CA 94115
(415) 923-3505
The Health and Healing Clinic is a specialty patient care center that integrates conventional medicine's knowledge and practice with appropriate complementary and alternative care. Under the auspices of California Pacific Medical Center's Institute for Health and Healing, the mission also includes rigorous scientific research of alternative modalities and continuing medical education. MDs with additional training and expertise in various alternative and complementary care modalities work in partnership with primary care physicians, specialists, and other care givers to provide patients with an integrated approach to their well being. Modalities include: Nutritional/Medicinal Therapies (diet, herbal, homeopathy), Energy Therapies (acupuncture, Yoga, Reiki), Somatic Therapies (physical manipulation, massage, bodywork), Spiritual Care (counseling and meditation), and Psychological support (mind/body medicine).

Health Enhancement Center
550 Water Street, Suite F4, Santa Cruz, CA
(408) 429-8046

Health Recovery Center
Joan Mathews-Larson, Ph.D.
E-mail: HRC@millcomm.com
3255 Hennepin Avenue South,
Minneapolis, MN 55408
(612) 827-7800; Fax (612) 827-1948

The Health Recover Center, a state licensed program for alcohol/drug addiction, has pioneered a holistic model of recovery that combines therapy with extensive bio-medical-nutritional repair.

Health Restoration Center
22706 Aspan Street, #501, Lake Forest, CA
(714) 770-9616

HealthEcology Therapy Center: The North Carolina School of the Healing Arts
Keith Bouchard, ND, Veronica Vela, ND
400 Oberlin Road, Suite 130, Raleigh, NC
(919) 832-8241; Fax (919) 468-0155
HealthEcology Therapy Center provides preventive and restorative health care services.
The North Carolina School of the Healing Arts is an educational curriculum in Natural Healing for individuals, families, professionals, and corporations.

Heights Chiropractic and Health Centre
4101 East Fourth Street, Long Beach, CA 90814
(562) 434-7260; Fax (562) 433-5058

Helios Health Center
4150 Darley Avenue, Suite 6, Boulder, CO
(303) 499-9224

Holistic Family Practice
4200 Westheimer, Houston, TX
(713) 626-0505

Holistic Health & Wellness Center
6615 North Atlantic Avenue, Cape Canaveral, FL
(407) 784-0930

Holistic Health Center
1505 Greenwood Road, Glenview, IL
(847) 486-0400

Holistic Medicine/Homeopathy
Edward S. Garbacz, MD
455 East Pace Ferry Road, Suite 201, Atlanta, GA
(404) 848-0033; Fax (404) 848-0438
Classical Homeopathy, nutritional medicine,
hormonal assessments (female, adrenal), digestive
evaluations, candida, food and environmental
allergies, integration with energetic methods
(Reiki, medical intuition) by referral.

Holistic Sports Medicine
1545 116th Northeast, Bellevue, WA
(206) 462-7433

House of Health
Box 459, Marshall, AR
(501) 448-3195

Institute for Mind Body Medicine
Dr. Benson
Deaconess Hospital, Deaconess Rd, Boston, MA 02215
(617) 632-9530

Institute of Human Potential
3901 Houma Boulevard, Suite 109, Metairie, LA
(504) 887-6270

Institute for Whole SpeCenterum Therapy
609 Walter Reed Drive, Greensboro, NC
(910) 292-1288

Kansas Longevity Center
707 Southeast Quincy, Suite 210, Topeka, KS
(913) 233-4650

Kerr House
17777 Beaver Street, Grand Rapids, OH
(419) 832-1733

Krieger Chiropractic Office
38-04 31st Avenue, Astoria, NY
(718) 726-0404

Live Oak Center for the Healing Arts
841 El Camino Real, Menlo Park, CA
(415) 323-4344

Magic Alive Now Healing Studio
Marcie Rose
4263 California Street, San Francisco, CA 94118
(415) 751-1782
Magic Alive Now Healing Studio creates an opportunity in which individuals may choose among a wide variety of holistic health modalities to enhance their unique healing process. The founder is certified in bodywork, rebirthing, counseling, dowsing, energy-work (Reiki and others), iridology, sclerology, meditation and nutrition. She also teaches private and small group healing classes and does a variety of spiritual counseling techniques. She focuses holistically to balance body, mind, emotions, and spirit by unblocking areas in peoples' lives that have prevented them from having what they want.

Marino Center for Progressive Health: Progressive Stress Reduction Program
Shreyes Patel, MD and Bill Chisholm
2500 Massachusetts Avenue, Cambridge, MA 02140
(617) 661-6225; Fax (617) 492-2002
An 8 week Mind/Body program incorporating mindful meditation and hatha yoga and other stress management techniques to help people cope with personal and professional stress and also chronic medical problems. Patients with chronic headaches, neck and low back pain, fibromyalgia, chronic fatigue syndrome, anxiety disorder, panic attacks, hypertension, diabetes, and insomnia participate in this program.

Mary's Place for Women & Their Families
400 Haber Road, Suite 401, Cary, IL
(708) 231-7750

Massage Professionals
28465 Front Street, Suite 221, Temecula, CA
(909) 695-1990

Medical Massage Center
Sue Jernigan RN, CNMT and assoc.
8370 West Coal Mine Avenue, Suite 106,
Littleton, CO 80128
(303) 979-0342; Fax (303) 979-3872
The staff of nationally certified professionals offer
neuromuscular therapy and therapeutic massage.
Each therapist has advanced training in the treatment
of acute and chronic pain. The center specializes in
muscular pain due to stress, injury, and pregnancy.
Causality Care Network. An increasing number of
insurers are covering our care.

Mind/Body Clinic at New England Deaconess Hospital:
Natural Healing Center, Inc.
243 Church Street Northwest, Suite 100 D, Vienna, VA
(703) 938-4868

Miro Center for Integrative Medicine
Connie Catellani, MD
1639 Orrington, Evanston, IL 60201
(847) 733-9900; Fax (847) 733-0105
The Miro Center for Healing is a physician directed
primary care facility with over 25 specialists in
traditional and non-traditional healing techniques.
The staff includes three physicians, an optometrist,
three psychologists, four acupuncturists, two
herbalists, three body workers, three energy workers,
two nutritionists, one homeopath, three nurse
practitioners, and one phlebotomist. The practitioners
treat all aspects of the patient: body, mind, and spirit.

Natural Medicine Clinic
104 East Sixth Avenue, Helena, MT
(406) 442-8508

Olive W. Garvey Center for Healing Arts
3100 North Hillside Street, Wichita, KS
(800) 447-7276

Options Center for Health & Education
4700 North Prospect, Road Suite A2,
Peoria Heights, IL
(309) 685-7721

Osmosis Enzyme Bath & Massage
www.osmosis.com
209 Bohemian Highway, Freestone, CA 95472
(707) 823-8231; Fax (707) 874-3788
Osmosis offers the deeply relaxing and rejuvenating
Japanese Enzyme Bath. You begin with tea in a rock
and water garden and are expertly cared for as you
take the bath and move onto the massage. The setting
is tranquil, serene, and surrounded by beautiful
gardens, 15 minutes from the Pacific Ocean.

Partners In Healing
900 Skokie Boulevard, Suite 100, Northbrook, IL 60062
(847) 509-8669
Partners in Healing is a holistic health center
dedicated to treating, educating, and empowering the
health care consumer and others seeking optimal
wellness in all life's arenas. Staffed by medical
doctors, nurses, chiropractors, podiatrist,
acupuncturist, naprapath, herbalists, nutritionists,
psychotherapists, and a non-denominational minister
who all work together, PIH is able to address the
whole you; body, mind, and spirit. Services include
acupuncture, aromatherapy, biofeedback, chiropractic,
energy balancing, Feldenkrais, guided imagery,
healing touch, herbology, homeopathy, hypnotherapy,
massage, meditation, naprapathy, massage,
nutritional, podiatry, psychoneurimmunology,
psychotherapy, soft tissue therapy, spiritual
counseling, sports psychology, support groups,
therapeutic exercise.

Partners In Wellness
Alyce Sorokie
1967 North Dayton, Chicago, IL 60614
(773) 868-4062
Colon Therapy, Nutritional Education, Therapeutic
Massage, Shiatsu, Holistic Counseling, Meditation
Classes, Dream Support Groups, Yoga, Gut Wisdom
classes/seminars..

Physical Medicine Clinic
5934 Royal Lane #250, Dallas, TX
(214) 890-7636

Portland Naturopathic Clinic
12231 Southeast Market Street, Portland, OR
(503) 255-7355

Preventive Medicine Associates
10700 Old County Road 15, Suite 350,
Minneapolis, MN
(612) 593-9458

Preventive Medicine Society
1000 Asylum Avenue, #2109, Hartford, CT
(203) 549-3444

Princeton Associates for Total Health
212 Commons Way, Princeton, NJ
(609) 921-1842

The Raj
1734 Jasmine Avenue, Fairfield, IA 52556
(515) 472-9580, (800) 248-9050; Fax (515) 472-2496
Ayurvedic treatments offered on a daily basis or as a
residential program.

Rees Family Medical Clinic
17308 Sunset Boulevard, Pacific Palisades, CA
(213) 454-5531

Reiki Training Institute
    Linda M. LaFlamme
    PO Box 481, Winchester, MA 01890
    (617) 729-3530; Fax (617) 721-7306
    The RTI is an internationally recognized teaching and
    resource center. We offer professional treatments and
    classes throughout the U.S. We support the Reiki
    community around the globe through classes,
    continuing education, products and services. We
    work closely with the medical community in
    providing Reiki treatments as a tool for patient health
    and wellness.

Rose Quest Nutrition Centre
    Chicago, IL
    (312) 444-9234
    Mishawaka, IN
    (219) 259-5653
    Rose Quest Nutrition Centre offers a system of
    nutrition which emphasizes personal responsibility
    and fosters a cooperative relationship between all
    those involved. Each person is viewed as a unique
    composition of physical, emotional, social, and
    spiritual dimensions, and total health requires the
    harmonious inner working of all these aspects.

Scottsdale Holistic Medical Group
    7350 East Stetson Drive, Suite 128, Scottsdale, AZ
    (602) 990-1528

Sedona Health & Wellness Center
    400 Soldiers Pass Road, Sedona, AZ
    (602) 282-2520

Shealy Institute
    1328 East Evergreen Street, Springfield, MO 65803
    (417) 865-5940
    As America's foremost center for alternative and
    holistic medicine, the Shealy Institute offers

comprehensive approaches to complex problems. Services available: comprehensive evaluations, complete examinations, diagnostic tests as needed, nutritional counseling, biofeedback training, habit control, lifestyle planning, TENS, therapeutic exercise, relaxation training, massage, acupuncture, computerized EEG brain mapping, comprehensive pain management (especially headache, back pain management, and depression), testing for brain injury, and cognitive retraining.

St. John Neuromuscular Pain Relief Institute
10950 72nd Street North, Suite 103, Largo, FL
(813) 541-1800

Stamford Pain Management Services
1290 Summer Street, Stamford, CT
(203) 961-1345

Stress Management
3930 Knowles Avenue, Suite 301, Kensington, MD
(301) 946-9334

Surfside Chiropractic
Dr. Lindsay Anglen
PO Box 221, Mount Vernon, MO 65712
(417) 466-7166; Fax (417) 466-7591
Holistic Nutritional Support, Chiropractic Care, Blood and Lab work, Acupuncture, and Diagnostics (EKG, X-ray, Spirometer, Doppler Ultrasound) and Qi-gong.

Synthesis Center
1507 Portage Street, Kalamazoo, MI
(616) 373-5600

Totalcare Medical Center
620 University Avenue, Palo Alto, CA
(415) 329-8001

Traditional Acupuncture Center
511 Main Street, Webster, SD
(605) 345-3344

Tree of Life Health Practice
Gabriel Cousens, MD
E-mail: tlrc@dakotacom.net
PO Box 778, Patagonia, AZ 85624
(520) 394-2060; Fax (520) 394-2099
This is a life-food, residential health and rejuvenation center in the mountains of Arizona where people may experience personal healing and develop a new lifestyle according to the body-mind-spirit ideas established in his three books. Dr. Cousens sees clients at the Center for health evaluations, medically supervised juice fasting, and Ayurvedic Pancha Karma cleansing.

Triad Health Practice
938 West Nelson, Chicago, IL
(312) 296-8400

Upledger Institute, Inc.: HealthPlex Clinical Services
E-mail: upledgeer@upledger.com
11211 Prosperity Farms Road, D325,
Palm Beach Gardens, FL 33410-3287
(561) 622-4706; Fax (561) 627-9231
UI HealthPlex provides individual appointments and intensive therapy programs based on Upledger Cranio Sacral Therapysm and SomatoEmotional Release(R). Other clinical services include acupuncture, hypnotherapy, psychotherapy and a range of manual therapies. UI is affiliated with the International Association of Healthcare Practitioners (IAHP). The Association's Directory, which is available for purchase, lists practitioners of manual therapies around the world.

Waveland Wellness Center
1346 West Waveland, Chicago, IL 60613
(312) 935-5050

Wellness Group
    Northbrook Court Professional Plaza, Suite 110,
    1535 Lake Cook Road, Northbrook, IL 60062
    (847) 559-9355

Wellness Potential, Inc.
    Cynthia Hrisco
    60 Overbrook Road, South Barrington, IL 60010
    (847) 842-1165; Fax (847) 842-1164
    Naturopathic, Homeopathic, Herbal Nutritional
    Therapies and laboratory testing. Applied
    Kinesiology, Adrenal profile (DHEA), Allergy and
    Antioxidant testing, Detoxification profile,
    Vitamin/Mineral assessment.

Wellness Unlimited
    6305 North Milwaukee, Chicago, IL
    (312) 775-2300

Whole Health Center
    5177 Richmond Avenue, #125, Houston, TX
    (713) 840-9355

Winter Haven Health Center: Chiropractic Neurology and
Sports Performance
    Dr. Nathan Conlee
    3020 North Country Club, Tucson, AZ 85716
    (520) 322-6161; Fax (520) 326-7716
    A Holistic approach to human performance using
    Performance Neurology, SuperHealth Nutrition,
    acupuncture, and more.

Women to Women
    Christiane Northrup, MD, FACOG
    1 Pleasant Street, Yarmouth, ME 04096
    (207) 846-6163

Healing Hospitals

Alegent Health System
Bergan-Mercy Medical Center
Omaha, NE
(402) 398-6040
A Planetree Affiliate.

Baptist Hospital
Center for Health and Wellness
Nashville, TN
(615) 284-6463
Programs for general stress-related disorders, Cardiac
Rehabilitation, Cardiac Risk Reduction, Chronic pain
and Healthy Lifestyles, a non-medical stress
management program.

Beth Israel Hospital
Picker/Commonwealth Program for
Patient-Centered Care
New York, NY
(212) 420-4247
A Planetree Affiliate.

California Pacific Medical Center
San Francisco, CA
(415) 561-1374
A Planetree Affiliate.

Cancer Treatment Centers of America
(800) 234-0497
Provides information about Hospitals with Cancer
Treatment Centers™ incorporating a whole person
approach. These Cancer Treatment Centers
incorporate a comprehensive approach integrating
advanced medical therapies with guided imagery,
relaxation, breathing techniques, natural food diets,
vitamin and mineral supplements, emotional support
and pastoral care. CTCA programs are located in

Midwestern Regional Medical Center in Zion, IL;
Cancer Treatment Center of Tulsa in Tulsa, OK; and
Maryview Medical Center in Portsmouth, VA.

Celebration Health
Orlando, FL
(407) 566-2400

Colorado Plains Medical Center
Fort Morgan, CO
(970) 867-3391
A Planetree Affiliate.

Columbia-Presbyterian Medical Center
Columbia Care Center, Department of Surgery
Jerry Whitworth, RN, C.C.P.
177 Fort Washington Avenue., MHB7 Room 435,
New York City, NY 10032
(212) 305-9628
On request, appointments for some alternative
therapies are made for patients in cardiology section.

Delano Regional Medical Center
Delano, CA
(805) 725-4800
A Planetree Affiliate.

Griffin Hospital
Derby, CT
(203) 732-7399
A Planetree Facility supporting patients in whole
healing (i.e. kitchens on every floor, arts and
entertainment programs).

Heart Disease Reversal Program
(203) 732-7410

Highland Hospital
Department of Medicine
Rochester, NY
(716) 473-2200

Highline Community Hospital
Seattle, WA
(206) 431-5304
A Planetree Affiliate.

Illinois Masonic Medical Center
Strong Spirit Wellness Center
938 West Nelson, Third Floor, Chicago, IL 60657
(773) 296-8410
Team of physicians, nurses, and alternative therapists
work cooperatively with you to customize services to
meet any special needs. Currently offering:
Acupuncture, Biofeedback, Guided Imagery,
Hawaiian Energetics, Integrative Structural
Bodywork, Massage Therapy, Meditation, Music
Therapy, Phoenix Rising Yoga Therapy,
Psychotherapy, Reiki, Shiastsu, Stress Management,
Support Groups, Tai Chi, and Yoga.

Kaiser Permanente
Vallejo Medical Center
Vallejo, CA
(707) 645-2101
Reportedly the first HMO-based alternative medicine
clinic. Patients can use acupuncture treatments for
pain management and take advantage of such
programs as relaxation training and nutritional
counseling.

Livingtson Foundation Medical Center
3232 Duke Street, San Diego, CA
(619) 224-3515

Marshall Hospital
Placerville, CA
(916) 622-1441
A Planetree Affiliate.

Maryview Medical Center
3636 High Street, Portsmouth, VA 23707
(804) 398-2064; Fax (804) 398-2070
Their medical center has a Cancer Treatment Centers
of America™ program.

Memorial Healthcare System
Mind/Body Medical Institute
Houston, TX
(713) 776-5020
Programs for general stress-related disorders,
infertility, Cardiac Rehabilitation, Cardiac Risk
Reduction, and Healthy Lifestyles, a non-medical
stress management program.

Mercy Hospital and Medical Center
2525 South Michigan Ave., Chicago, IL 60616
(312) 567-2600
Less Stress, a five week stress management program;
Wellspace program (Feldenkrais Method, Meditation
Instruction, Zero Balancing). Complementary
medicine program beginning to be incorporated into
medical care (ie healing music in Intensive Care).

Mid-Columbia Medical Center
The Dalles, OR
(541) 296-1111
A Planetree Affiliate.

Midwestern Regional Medical Center
Zion, IL 60099
(847) 872-4561, (800) 765-9920
Cancer patients can access massage and creative
visualization sessions. The cancer program is
managed by Cancer Treatment Centers of America™.

Morristown Memorial Hospital
Mind/Body Medical Institute
Morristown, NJ
(201) 971-4575

Programs for general stress-related disorders, Cancer and Infertility Programs, and Healthy Lifestyles, a non-medical stress management program.

New York University Medical Center
Co-op Care
(212) 263-7300

Pacific Presbyterian Hospital
2351 Clay Street, Suite 322, San Francisco, CA
(415) 923-3696

Parkland Memorial Hospital
Dallas City Hospital District
(817) 590-8131

Peekskill Area Health Center
Peekskill, NY
(914) 734-8800
A Planetree Affiliate.

Riverside Methodist Hospital
Mind/Body Medical Institute
Columbus, OH
(614) 566-4050
Programs for general stress-related disorders, Chronic pain and Healthy Lifestyles, a non-medical stress management program.

Rush Presbyterian-St. Luke's Medical Center
Chicago, IL
(312) 942-5000
Have a (cancer) unit that is patient-focused, supporting holistic approaches.

Samaritan Health System
Phoenix, AZ
(602) 495-4000
A Planetree Affiliate.

Scripps Clinic Wellness Program
Alisa Miniar
10666 North Torrey Pines Road, La Jolla, CA
(619) 554-8835; Fax (619) 554-4065
Health education and health promotion programs
including: Nutrition counseling, Weight management,
Stress management, Asthma education, Prenatal
education, Cardiovascular health, Smoking cessation,
Diabetes education, Spinal health.

Shawano Community Hospital
Shawano, WI
(715) 526-2111
A Planetree Affiliate.

St. Joseph's Hospital Regional Cancer Center
1100 West Steward Drive, Orange, CA
(714) 771-8938

St. Mary's Hospital
Amsterdam, NY
(518) 842-1900

St. Peter's Medical Center
New Brunswick, NJ
(908) 745-8528
Programs for general stress-related disorders and
Healthy Lifestyles, a non-medical stress management
program.

Stratton VA Medical Center
Albany, NY
(518) 462-6069
A Planetree Affiliate.

University of Arizona
(520) 626-5077

University of Massachusetts Medical Center
  Stress Reduction Clinic
  Carol Lewis
  Worcester, MA
  (508) 856-2656

University of Texas Health Science Center
  Rehabilitation Science
  Dallas, TX
  (972) 883-2747

Wellness Center/Grant Hospital of Chicago
  550 West Webster, Chicago, IL
  (312) 883-3777

Wellness Medical Institute
  Edward A. Taub
  1001 North Tustin Avenue, Santa Ana, CA 92705
  (800) 720-9355

Healing Retreats/Spas

A Touch of Wellness
654 Van Loo Road, Canon City, CO
(719) 269-1912

Commonweal Cancer Help Retreat
PO Box 316, Bolinas, CA 94924
(415) 868-0970
Offers retreats for people seeking physical, mental,
emotional, and spiritual healing in the face of cancer.
(*From Choices in Healing: Integrating the Best of
Conventional and Complementary Approaches to
Cancer*, by Michael Lerner).

The Cooper Aerobics Center
12230 Preston Road, Dallas, TX 75230
(214) 386-4777, (800) 444-5192; Fax (214) 386-0039
Programs supporting life-style changes.

Duke University Diet and Fitness Center
804 West Trinity Avenue, Durham, NC 27701
(919) 684-6331, (800) 362-8446; Fax (919) 682-8869
Programs supporting lifestyle changes.

Eden Valley Lifestyle Center
Daniel D. McKibben and Carol Bearce
105522.761@compuserve.com
6263 North Country Road #29, Loveland, CO 80538
(800) 637-WELL, (970) 669-7730; Fax (970) 667-1742
Our Lifestyle Center, staffed with a physician, hydro
and massage therapies, offers natural healing to body,
mind and spirit. The Center is primarily an
educational program. Guests come from 1-3 weeks.
The program includes hydrotherapy treatments
(sauna, Jacuzzi, hydrocollators), massage, physical
exam, health consultations, exercises, walks, a vegan
diet, natural health classes/demonstrations and
cooking schools. The program has proved successful

for many of the following conditions: weight management, smoking cessation, arthritis, diabetes and hypoglycemia, degenerative diseases, allergies, heart problems, stroke recovery and prevention, and high blood pressure.

Filhoa Meadows
14628 Highway 133, Redstone, CO 81623
(970) 963-1989, (800) 227-8906
Health retreat.

Foxhollow Wellness Spa
Route 7, Lenox, MA 01240
(800) 282-5212, (413) 637-2000

The Greenbrier
White Sulphur Springs, WV 24986
(304) 536-1110, (800) 624-6070; Fax (304) 536-7854
Health examinations allow for the combination of diagnostic and preventive medicine with the spa experience.

Hartland Wellness Center
Box 1, Rapidan, VA 22733
(540) 672-3100, (800) 763-9355; Fax (540) 672-2584
Wellness Programs.

Hilton Head Health Institute
Box 7138, Hilton Head Island, SC 29938
(803) 785-7292, (800) 292-2440; Fax (803) 686-5659
A program emphasizing behavior modification.

Himalayan Institute and Publishers
RR1, Box 400, Honesdale, PA
(800) 822-4547

Maharishi Ayur-Veda Health Center
679 George Hill Road, Box 344, Lancaster, MA 01523
(508) 365-4549; Fax (508) 368-0674
Residential Ayurvedic treatments.

Meadowlark
    26126 Fairview Avenue
    (714) 927-1343

Pritikin Longevity Center
    1910 Ocean Front Walk, Santa Monica, CA 90405
    (310) 450-5433, (800) 421-9911; Fax (310) 450-3602
    5875 Collins Avenue, Miami Beach, FL 33140
    (305) 866-2237, (800) 327-4914; Fax (305) 866-1872
    Medically supervised programs supporting healthy
    lifestyles. Designed for healthy people who want to
    learn how to maintain their health as well as for
    people with certain chronic conditions.

St. Helena Hospital Health Center
    Deer Park, CA 94576
    (707) 963-6200, (800) 358-9195
    Offers residential health enhancement programs, and
    the McDougall (diet and nutrition) program.

Weimer Institute
    Box 486, 20601 West Paoli Lane, Weimer, CA 95736
    (916) 637-4111, (800) 525-9192
    Residential health enhancement programs.

Wildwood Lifestyle Center
    Box 129, Wildwood, GA 30757
    (706) 820-1490, (800) 634-9355; Fax (706) 820-1474
    Teaches participants healthier ways of life.

Appendix

I. _Looking for the Right Practitioner_

Choosing the right practitioner for you is a subjective process. Ask your friends and colleagues if they use any alternative practitioners and who they would recommend. Whether or not you have referrals to a practitioner, you might ask one you are considering if you could speak with him/her about their practice to help you decide if you would like to use them. Have this checklist with you when you speak with a practitioner to help you decide if this is someone who you want on your wellness team.

- Are you comfortable with the practitioner, and do you feel comfortable asking questions?
- Does the practitioner listen to you or does s/he have his/her mind somewhere else?
- Do you feel welcome in their office? Do people seem to be conscientious and caring?
- Do you get the sense that they have good quality care and administrative processes to support the care given?
- Do you understand what would be required of you in the healing process, and is this something you are willing to participate in?

II. _Meeting with Your Practitioner_

Remember when you meet with your practitioner that you are the focus of attention. You do not need to feel intimidated by the practitioner or their staff – they are there to help you. I strongly suggest you **write your questions and concerns down before the visit** so you remember everything you want to talk about. You might ask:

- Explain my condition.
- What are my treatment options?
- What are the potential side effects?
- When do I need to make my decision, and what are the consequences of delaying a decision?

- What can I do to help myself?
- Follow up with any issues that are left incomplete and keep good notes between visits as well as during your visits.

III. *Finding a Holistic Hospital*

Here are some points you may consider when looking for a holistic, patient-focused hospital.

- Are the visiting hours liberal (can family/friends visit 24 hours)?
- Do they serve healthy food? Ask the nutritionist if they cook with grains and whole foods.
- Are the cleaning supplies non-toxic? What can they tell you about their ventilation and filtration systems?
- Ask about their quality assurance programs, and ask what kind of data they collect. Do you feel they care about customer satisfaction?
- What kind of education is available to patients and their families?
- What kind of complementary/alternative/adjunct approaches are available to patients?

IV. *Keeping Track of Your Health Visits*

When you are seeing multiple physicians and holistic providers it is important to keep your "team" of providers current on what the others are doing. You are the common link between them, and if you take responsibility for educating them about your case you are more likely to receive appropriate care. Keep a notebook for recording the following valuable information.

Date of Visit
Provider Name
Tests
Results/Recommendations
Medication/Supplements

— Notes —

— Notes —

— Notes —

— Notes —

— Notes —

— Notes —

— Notes —

— Notes —

— Notes —

— Notes —

— Notes —

— Notes —

References

Benson, Herbert. *The Relaxation Response.* New York: Avon Publishing, 1975.

Brennan, Barbara. *Hands of Light.* New York: Bantam Doubleday Dell Publishing Group, Inc., 1993.

Burt, Bernard. *Fodor's Healthy Escapes.* New York: Fodor's Travel Publication, Inc., 1997.

Chopra, Deepak. *Perfect Health.* New York: Harmony Books, 1991.

Clayton and McCullough, Virginia. *A Consumers Guide to Alternative Health Care.* Holbrook, MA: Adams Publishing, 1995.

Cousins, Norman. *Anatomy of an Illness.* New York: Bantam Books, 1979.

Dossey, Barbara. "Using Imagery to Help Your Patient Heal". *American Journal of Nursing.* June 1995; 41-47.

Dossey, Larry. *Healing Words: The Power of Prayer and the Practice of Medicine.* San Francisco: Harper Collins, 1993.

Dossey, Larry. *Prayer is Good Medicine: How to Reap the Healing Benefits of Prayer.* San Francisco: Harper, 1996.

Eisenberg DM, Kessler RC, Foster C, et al. "Unconventional medicine in the United States: prevalence, costs and patterns of use". *New England Journal of Medicine* 1993, 328: 246-52.

Fugh-Berman, Adriane, *Alternative Medicine: What Works.* Tucson: Odonian Press, 1996.

Good, Marion. "Relaxation Techniques for Surgical Patients". *American Journal of Nursing.* May 1995; 39-43.

Goleman, Daniel, Ph.D. and Joel Gurin. *Mind Body Medicine.* Yonkers, New York: Consumer Reports Books, 1993.

Kabat-Zinn, Jon. *Full Catastrophe Living: Using the Wisdom of Your Body and Mind to Face Stress, Pain and Illness.* New York: Delacorte Press, 1990

Kabat-Zinn, Jon, Lipworth L, Burney R, Sellers W. 'Four year follow-up of a meditation-based program for the self-regulation of chronic pain: treatment outcomes and compliance'. *Clinical Journal of Pain* 1986; 159-73.

Kabat-Zinn J, Massion AO, Kristeller J, et al. 'Effectiveness of a meditation-based stress reduction program in the treatment of anxiety disorders'. *American Journal of Psychiatry* 1992; 149(7):936-43.

Keegan, Lynn. 'Nurses are Embracing Holistic Healing'. *RN* April 1996; 59-60.

Kornfeld, Hulen S. 'Co-Meditation: Guiding patients through the relaxation process'. *RN* Nov. 1995; 57-59.

Krieger, Dolores. *The Therapeutic Touch: How to Use Your Hands to Help or Heal.* Englewood Cliffs, NJ: Prentice-Hall, 1979.

Laskow, Leonard, MD. *Healing With Love.* New York: HarperSanFrancisco, 1992.

Ledwith, Stuart P. 'Therapeutic touch and mastectomy: A case study'. *RN* July 1995; 51-53.

Leviton, Richard. 'Healing Vibrations'. *Yoga Journal* Jan.-Feb. 1994; 59-126.

Mackey, Rochelle B. 'Discover the Healing Power of Therapeutic Touch'. *American Journal of Nursing.* April 1995; 27-33.

Meintz, Sharon L. 'Whatever became of the backrub?' *RN* April 1995; 49-56.

Nhat Hahn, Thich. *The Miracle of Mindfulness: A Manual on Meditation.* New York: Beacon Press, 1975.

Northrup, Christine. *Women's Bodies: Women's Wisdom.* New York: Bantam Books, 1994.

Ornish, Dean. *Stress, Diet and Your Heart.* New York: NAL Dutton, 1984.

Rossman, Martin. *Healing Yourself: A Step-by-Step Program for Better Health Through Imagery.* New York: Simon & Schuster, 1987.

Schmidt, Carol M. 'The basics of therapeutic touch'. *RN* June 1995; 50-54.

Schulte, Evie. 'Acupuncture: Where East Meets West'. *RN* Oct. 1996; 55-57.

Selby, Anna. Aromatherapy. New York: Macmillan, 1996.

Shames, Karilee Halo. 'Harness the Power of Guided Imagery'. *RN* Aug. 1996; 49-50.

Shealy, Norman. *The Complete Family Guide to Alternative Medicine*. New York: Barnes and Noble Books, Inc., 1996.

Shinkarovsky, Louisa. 'Hypnotherapy-not just hocus pocus'. *RN* June 1996; 55-57.

Siegel, Bernie S. *Peace, Love and Healing*. New York: Harper & Row, Publishers, 1989.

Simonton, Carl. *Healing into Life*.

Swackhamer, Annette H. 'It's Time to Broaden our Practice'. *RN* Jan .1995; 49-51.

Tatton, Cynthia Wright. 'Touch of all kinds - is therapeutic'. *RN* Feb. 1996; 61-64.

Van Sell, Sharon L. 'Reiki: An Ancient Touch Therapy'. *RN* Feb. 1996; 57-59.

Weil, Andrew. *Natural Health, Natural Medicine*. New York: Houghton Mifflin Company, 1995.

Weil, Andrew. *Spontaneous Healing: How to Discover and Enhance Your Body's Natural Ability to Maintain and Heal Itself*. New York: Alfred A. Knopf, 1995.

Weil, Andrew. *8 Weeks to Optimum Health*. New York: Alfred A Knopf, Inc., 1997.

Worwood, Valerie Ann. *The Fragrant Mind*. Novato, CA: New World Library, 1996.

Index

Contact Submission Form

We love hearing about people and places that support the integration of holistic and conventional health practices. Please send us:

- Name, Address, Phone & Fax information for each organization/program
- Contact person
- Description of programs/services
- Type of Entry: Association, Research Organization/Service, Educational Organization/Program, Health Insurance, Publication, Web site, Healing Clinic/Center, Hospital, Retreat/Spa.

Thank-You!

> EMPR
> PO Box 14684
> Chicago, IL 60614-0684

Order & Communication Form

Visit our Web Page: www.healthy-solutions-us.com

Where to Go When You're Hurting:
A Healing Resource Guide

We hope this book has been useful to you. Your comments are welcome, and may find themselves in future editions of this book! You can contact us by e-mail at EMPR@pobox.com, or drbeth@ibm.net, by phone at (888) 302-8248 or by using our mailing address.

This book is available for $19.95 plus $3 shipping and handling (please add 8.75% tax, which is $1.75 per book, for shipments to Illinois). To order additional books, send your name, address, and phone number along with your check or money order to:

EMPR
PO Box 14684
Chicago, IL 60614-0684

Thanks, and best wishes for good health!

- -

Name:_____

Address:_____

City, State, Zip:_____

Phone:_____

Quantity @ $19.95 _____

Subtotal: _____

For Illinois delivery add 8.75% sales tax _____

Shipping and Handling, $3 per book _____

Total: _____

Order & Communication Form

Visit our Web Page: www.healthy-solutions-us.com

Where to Go When You're Hurting:
A Healing Resource Guide

We hope this book has been useful to you. Your comments are welcome, and may find themselves in future editions of this book! You can contact us by e-mail at EMPR@pobox.com, or drbeth@ibm.net, by phone at (888) 302-8248, or by using our mailing address.

This book is available for $19.95 plus $3 shipping and handling (please add 8.75% tax, which is $1.75 per book, for shipments to Illinois). To order additional books, send your name, address, and phone number along with your check or money order to:

EMPR
PO Box 14684
Chicago, IL 60614-0684

Thanks, and best wishes for good health!

- -

Name:_____

Address:_____

City, State, Zip:_____

Phone:_____

Quantity @ $19.95 _____

Subtotal: _____

For Illinois delivery add 8.75% sales tax _____

Shipping and Handling, $3 per book _____

Total: _____

Order & Communication Form

Visit our Web Page: www.healthy-solutions-us.com

Where to Go When You're Hurting: A Healing Resource Guide

We hope this book has been useful to you. Your comments are welcome, and may find themselves in future editions of this book! You can contact us by e-mail at EMPR@pobox.com, or drbeth@ibm.net, by phone at (888) 302-8248, or by using our mailing address.

This book is available for $19.95 plus $3 shipping and handling (please add 8.75% tax, which is $1.75 per book, for shipments to Illinois). To order additional books, send your name, address, and phone number along with your check or money order to:

> **EMPR**
> **PO Box 14684**
> **Chicago, IL 60614-0684**

Thanks, and best wishes for good health!

Name:_____

Address:_____

City, State, Zip:_____

Phone:_____

Quantity @ $19.95 _____

Subtotal: _____

For Illinois delivery add 8.75% sales tax _____

Shipping and Handling, $3 per book _____

Total: _____